The Fertile
FIZZ

The Kickstarter Special Edition

Thank you

To all the fine folk who supported our campaign,
you put your pledges where our heart is

This first edition is dedicated to each and everyone of you

The Fertile
FIZZ

Jani White

Artwork by Carolyn Weltman
Poetry by Rebecca Deacon

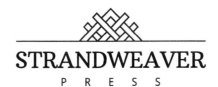

STRANDWEAVER
P R E S S

Published by Strandweaver Press

Text © 2016 Jani White
Original artwork by Carolyn Weltman. All rights reserved
Original poetry HIM & HER © Rebecca Deacon and The Gypsy Pirate. All rights reserved

The right of Jani White to be identified as author of this Work has been asserted by him/her in accordance with sections 77 and 78 of the Copyright, Designs and Patents Act 1988

ISBN 978-0-9935838-0-3

A CIP catalogue record for this book is available from the British Library

Cover design: Clare Turner

Typesetting: Megan Sheer

Publishing Consultants: Heather Boisseau & Clare Christian at RedDoor Publishing

Printed and bound by CPI Group (UK) Ltd, Croydon, CR0 4YY

Contents

Foreword
By Dr Jane Lyttleton

I am pleased to be able to introduce a completely different sort of book into the plethora of fertility self-help books that we see on the shelves these days. And *The Fertile Fizz* certainly is different – it asks the reader to go back to their primal selves, back to where we were before we all became so 'post-modern' (and drowned in busyness and technology).

I talk about sex a lot in my clinic – about the hows, whens and wherefores – well mostly the whens, occasionally the hows. And although I am, like the author of this book, guilty of occasionally suggesting breaking the no-alcohol rule for would-be mothers, to encourage a mid-cycle tryst with a tipple, I have to admit the word Fizz has been lacking from the conversation. My patients and I joke about 'baby-sex' and the well-known slogan 'just do it' … but often it's more with a sigh of resignation rather than it is with a spark of inspiration.

The question, 'HOW do we keep having sex over and over, month after month, year after year?' that couples who have been trying to conceive a long time ask, is an important one that is seldom addressed. But here is a book that not only talks about bringing the spark back to baby-sex – but talks about it from every angle – hormonally, neurologically and erotically.

Jani White calls this the Fizz. The Brazilians have a good word for it too – 'Tezao' (pronounced something like tezaaung). It refers to something or someone particularly exciting and pleasant (though nowadays in street slang it has lost some of its poetry and refers merely to an erection).

This book contains some important messages – important because no one else is saying this – the assisted fertility and IVF clinics certainly don't! I mean, have you heard them talking about 'Yang Wilt'? These messages might be confronting to some couples, especially those who have turned to IVF and have relegated sex (let alone Fizz) to the back burner. But Jani uses quirky humour to make a serious matter (not conceiving) into a fun matter (spicing up the bedroom) and provides compelling reasons for couples to stay engaged with the process.

We know now from functional MRI studies that love and desire are not so much emotions but they are actually drives from a more primitive part of the brain. It all starts with puberty and the production of oestrogen and testosterone, the first and most basic hormonal drivers for lust. Then when we meet that special someone who is particularly attractive to us, and feel the 'Tezao' or 'Fizz', dopamine floods our brains and we are in love – or a state of limerence to use the technical (but still quite romantic) word. Palpitations, euphoria and walking on air characterise this stage, sexual desire and Fizz are NOT lacking. This crazy and addictive stage of the mating game is highly adaptive for reproducing but in modern society it seldom coincides with the right time to have a baby – there is more study to be done, the career ladder to be climbed, travel to be experienced, the mortgage to be faced… so many things to tick off the list first before babies.

And such a high-tension state of attraction can't last… two years at the most. So when a couple finally gets around to thinking it's the right time to start a family, the necessary baby-making activity can actually become a chore, flat with no Fizz… and when becoming pregnant takes a bit longer than expected, the situation goes from bad to worse.

This is the very sad state of affairs that Jani White addresses in her book. She advises couples to focus on cultivating oxytocin production, the cuddle and bonding hormone, to rekindle that chemistry of attraction so that it becomes the chemistry of conception, and libido once again becomes the power behind conception.

Jani reminds her patients to keep coming back to that important choice made in the early heady days of falling in love when the initial rush of dopamine led you to choose each other, to bond and become each other's mate and partner.

But in addition to the chemistry of attraction, Jani also talks about important factors like Imagination, Patience and Receptivity. And on the other side of the coin, she talks about how to manage Stress, Angst, Hope and Fear. The book finishes with some wise words about pacing ourselves, gentle exercise, good food and cultivating Vitality. Much of this wisdom springs from the well of Traditional Chinese Medicine. Good advice for everyone!

Jani sprinkles her biology and neurology lessons with erotic Lautrecian bordello images of wasp-waisted women and their hunky partners to feed the inner fantasy worlds of her readers. Indeed, there is something here for everyone!

Dr Jane Lyttleton
Sydney, Australia
April 2016

Introduction

In 1968, when I was 6 years old and my brothers were 2 and 4, my mother lost her fourth child, our little sister Susan. She was taken away from my mother at birth, at a time when fathers were still not allowed into the labour room, and neither of my parents were ever allowed to see her. My mother came home from the hospital a mere 3 days later, and she fell into a place of utter desolation. At the time, Susan's death was dealt with by pretending as if nothing had happened. There wasn't even a funeral.

We not only lost my sister, we also lost my mother to a profound depression, we lost my father to his workaholic/alcoholic demise, and as a unit our family never quite fully recovered from the impact of Susan's death.

It's nearly half a century since this happened and I'm glad to say that there has been a profound change in our society. What we experienced as a family in the 1960s would be highly unlikely to occur within the health care provision of today.

This is why I do the work I do. The impact of losing my sister, of experiencing my parent's grief – experiencing all the mistakes, the lack of appropriate care, that led to the splinters and shards they never recovered from – this has been the driving force of my life. This is the reason why my fertility practice, and my work as a doula, as an antenatal teacher, and as an acupuncturist is all based in helping people to have healthy babies, to become happy families.

Funnily enough, I never actually set out to have a fertility practice. It was always all about obstetrics for me. Recently qualified and just starting up my pregnancy practice, my colleague Sharyn Singer, a nutritionist, began to send me her difficult fertility cases. It did not take us long to realise the combination of Input (nutrition) and Uptake (acupuncture) was a very winning combination, and before we knew it our fertility work took off of its own accord.

In the 17 years that I have been working with couples who are trying to conceive I have felt the ANGST of your fears and shared the joys when that longed for pregnancy occurs. I guess you can say, due to the experiences of my childhood, I have a finely tuned radar for the wobble factor, and perhaps people who come to my clinic space realise – here is a safe port to be able to unpack the difficult bits. This heart-felt sharing is what informs my words.

And so this book is all about those hard to cope with emotions that accompany this journey to conceive. It is coupled with risqué cheerfulness and plenty of advice of all the good things you CAN do. It is invested with the intention to help you find your own way forward within the challenges you are facing.

At the core of conceiving is the lovemaking that you share, for it is your sexual attraction that *is* the very base line of conception. Throughout the writing of the *Fertile Fizz*, it was ever in my mind's eye that this book should be seeded with erotic images and prose. The things that excite us derive from our *imagination*, and I wanted to bring something tangible to this book to entice and excite your sensual and sexual longings.

Between each chapter I bring you the stimulating poems of Rebecca Deacon, whose soul-bearing words are perfectly embraced by the voluptuous images of fine artist Carolyn Weltman. Their work encapsulates the joys of exploration and the heartfelt tenderness between lovers.

These images and poems are authentic – real people, real connection, real intimacy – the spirit of sexuality they exude imbibes this book with the essence that I wish for you to experience with each other; seeking to find connection within the vulnerability, to find the bravery to tackle the issues that are clouding your intimacy.

My wish is that you may flow towards the authenticity between you, to open into your own sexuality with all of the emotional connection and physical delight that is at the very heart of conceiving.

The chemistry of attraction *is* the chemistry of conception.

X jw

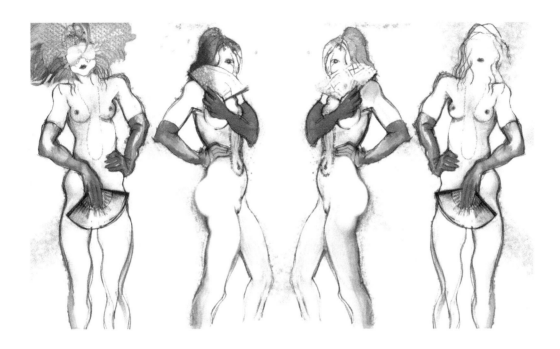

How to use this book

This book is essentially a very sexy biology lesson

The reasons we might not be conceiving crosses a very wide spectrum; each one of you has a unique profile of the things that are impediments, difficulties and challenges within your own unique circumstances.

This book is designed for you to dip in and choose, to connect with the things that are meaningful for you, and to cherry pick the bits that may help you towards finding your own way forward.

Modern life is stressful, and the advice seeded throughout this text is aimed at helping you understand a) the chemistry of how stress interferes with conception, and b) how you can actually change the stress impact and improve your receptivity to conceive.

The *Fertile Fizz* is about so much more than coping with the emotional difficulties, it is about understanding how all of your systems orchestrate together to help aid conception.

We don't just get pregnant with our gynaecology, we get pregnant with our whole bodies: our gynae, our digestion, our hearts and our minds. The road to good health, and to healthy conception, is paved with good intestines. This book will give you a much clearer understanding of how diet and nutrition affect your sexuality and reproduction, and will inspire you to really understand how much the way you eat affects your libido, which is your pathway to conception.

And so dear reader, sally forth, and find your way, the way that is your own way. Enjoy the hot sexy bits, and, if reading this book becomes yet another stress, then please just put it down. This book is to support you, help you to feel positive and to ignite your sense of sexuality within the context of trying to conceive.

Enjoy!

PS There is a glossary of English idioms in the endnotes for any of the words or phrases that may flummox you …

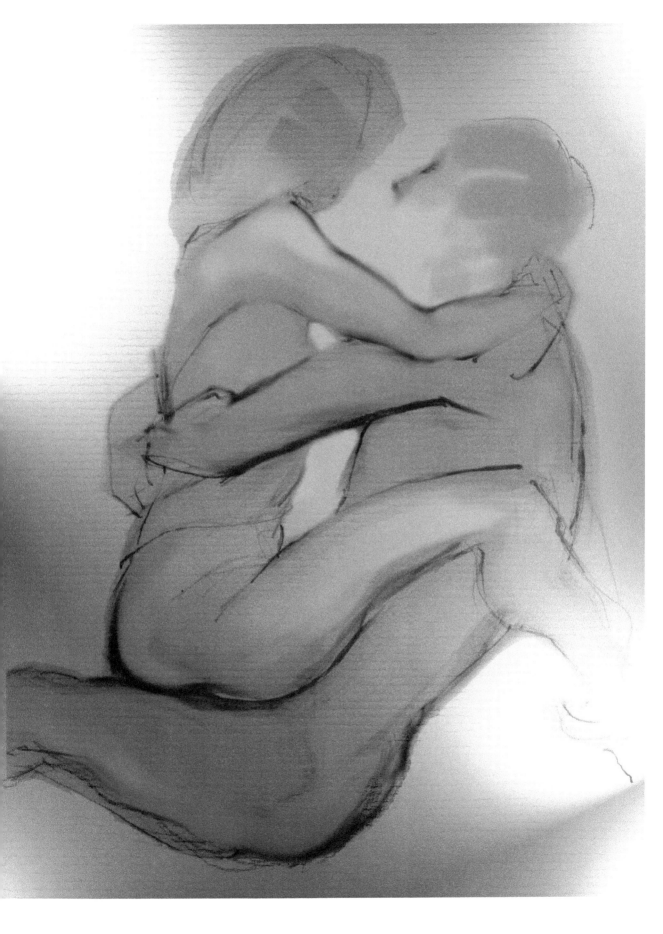

Chapter One

Bubbly Fizz

I got a phone call the other day from my colleague Michael Dooley, a renowned fertility consultant, who demanded of me: 'Jani White! What on earth is this advice I hear you are giving to our patients? Why in heaven's name are you suggesting that it is OK to drink alcohol – you know how hard we work to get across the message to avoid alcohol when women are trying to conceive!!' (He really does speak with all these exclamation marks.)

I laughed, for the level of outrageous indignation was delivered with Michael's rather splendid Irish humour. With a corresponding chuckle I threw on my own most equally pseudo-posh voice: 'But Michael – I am not recommending just any alcohol! I am recommending champagne!! (I too speak with exclamation marks.) Bubbles of deliciousness that bring you into a lovely uplifted happy lightness – with champagne you don't have to get drunk, you get floaty …

'Our TTC (trying-to-conceive) couples are working hard enough already. They are doing everything they know to be right: no alcohol, no caffeine, no drugs, no cigarettes, no toxins, preservatives or additives; they are constantly controlling their diets, as organic as possible, often with restrictions of wheat, dairy and sugar, they are taking supplements or choking down their Chinese herbs, no laptops on the groin or phones in the pocket, they've given up the Y-fronts and the cycling, they are changing work habits, doing their yoga and reflexology and seeing an acupuncturist, and goodness knows absolutely anyone else whom they believe may be able to help them …

'Then there may be the scary gamut of fertility testing, the mill of finding their way through the medical systems, waiting for appointments and test results, and struggling through the maze of investigations into fertility treatment, or finding themselves barrelling down an IVF track they did not expect, worried if they can afford it ...

'Even worse, they can be left in the no-man's land of "unexplained infertility", even though all their fertile markers are in normal range they are being told they have infertility, a most confusing and disheartening analysis that does not actually amount to an actual diagnosis ...

'All the while, they are busy charting, taking temperatures every morning, recording mucus changes, peeing on LH test strips for days on end, watching the clock, timing the intercourse, feeling the pressure of trying to take advantage of the right timings, all in the context of the regular grind of everyday work commitments ...

'Not to mention the whole 2 weeks of waiting through the luteal phase [post ovulation, where fertilisation may occur] to see if maybe, just maybe, oh please God let it happen this month. All the while assessing every twinge – is this implantation or just premenstrual pain? – and waiting and waiting and waiting – only to bleed again, crying the sorrow while trying to find the courage to start the whole damn process all over again …

'Trying to conceive can become a full time all-consuming litany of thou shall not do this and thou shall only do that ...

'So what I'm recommending Michael is that they keep a nice chilled bottle of bubbly in the fridge, and when the stretchy mucus or LH surge appears there is a happy treat awaiting them. On that special day they can text their lover "hey baby, come on home early tonight", then get out the sexy lingerie, light a few candles, share the bubbly, and in the joyful glow of that golden effervescence, shag each other senseless for the sheer fun of it!'

There was a very long pause, and our Michael simply replied: 'Ahh, I think I should quite like to borrow that advice!'

NB: If you don't like champagne, anything that gives you Fizz will do – a favourite beer, a nice chilled white, a deep full-bodied sexy velvety red. If that doesn't float your boat perhaps a Fizzy gin and tonic or such will, but please be mindful that spirits have a much higher alcohol content, and it is detrimental to your fertility to drink regularly or to actually get drunk.

If you are teetotal – great for your fertility – then choose something you really think of as a treat, perhaps an elderflower cordial with fresh lemon and a sprig of mint (in a champagne flute of course!). Any drink that feels special and different is the idea. When you are working so very hard and on so very many levels to conceive, then at that 'tenterhooks' time of ovulation I would like to advocate a treat, as long as it it's in moderate quantity and of excellent quality. (Now that should make Michael happy ...)

The Fertile Fizz

This book is all about what happens when we first see that certain someone, and, catching their eye and reading that certain glint, we think: 'Cor yeah baby, I'd like to shag you.'

That is the Fizz – a chemical reaction – unbidden, primal, an urge, instinct, intuition – whereby the pheromones have signalled to the limbic system and the dopamine flows, kicking off the oxytocin – and well beyond our cognitive reasoning or choice, we fall into attraction.

Part of what is happening is that the pheromonal signalling has told the brain, here are genes that will mix well with ours: this is a person we should mate with. The primal drive to procreate is not something that we choose, it is hardwired into our DNA – the DNA that flavours the tone, timbre, vibrancy, resonance and smell of our pheromones – magical antennae that tell us who is a good genetic match and when it's time to do the dirty.

The chemistry of attraction is the primary driver for procreation, and hormonally we are structured to respond to that limbic messaging of desire. The chemistry of our sexuality is predicated on that attraction factor. It is the chemistry of our sexuality that constructs, underpins and enhances the chemistry of conception.

In the throes of trying-to-conceive (TTC) many (most – err – virtually all) couples will experience some sense of imposition or drain upon their intimacy, as the scheduling of sperm delivery begins to drive the sex, pressuring uncomfortable sexual politics into the frame of a couple's relationship. The fun often goes out of the lovemaking, and is very often replaced by sex-with-an-agenda.

The Fizz that can be triggered when a couple's eyes first meet is exactly the same Fizz that brings sperm and egg into attraction. The more someone is in their oxytocin state, the more receptive the body becomes, generating a welcoming conducive atmosphere for fertilisation and implantation. In this book I want to address just why it is so important to keep our focus and energy within the sphere of desire, for it is attraction that initiates the Fizz.

But Trying To Conceive is stressful. And the longer it goes on, the more core-shakingly awful it can become. For many TTC couples the burden of trying to live through their daily stresses and still find the energy to ignite their sexuality, in the face of the stress hormones shutting down the desire hormones, creates a conflict between heart and mind that affects both body and soul. We will look at practical ways in which you can address these stresses to radically change your approach to trying to conceive.

This book is designed to help you understand the chemistry of attraction – essentially the chemistry of conception – and how the stress response can interfere with your attraction and conception cascades.

My ambition is to show you how, through understanding the chemical Fizz of your endocrine (your hormone management systems) you will be greatly empowered to manage your Fizz into a place where the stress does not have to block your pathway to conception.

This book is essentially a very sexy biology lesson.

Oxytocin Fizz

When we look at conception in this context of cascading hormones, the simplest thing to understand is that if you are in the parasympathetic aspect of your autonomic nervous system (don't worry! I'll explain in more detail), then it is possible for the oxytocin to flow.

If the oxytocin can flow, this can lead to orgasm. Having orgasm will lead to more oxytocin. For a woman, having an orgasm is the finest way to facilitate conception, generating the movement of lots of blood into the pelvic muscles, stimulating the exchange and flow of energies throughout the pelvic region and the reproductive organs, bringing a powerful sperm delivery right up against the cervix, and causing the cervix to dip and gulp (really! more on this later ...). Not to mention that orgasm just feels so good!

The best possible way to make babies is in lovemaking that is all about enjoying sex, loving your lover, being loved, turning each other on. This is at the core of what this book is all about.

Do you remember what it was like when you first met? When you wanted to spend hours just kissing because it just felt so good? All that delicious eye contact and hand holding … When you stepped through the door and started tearing each other's clothes off the very second the door closed. When you would go to bed at 7 p.m. because a night under the duvet together was more fun than any movie or outing could possibly be.

This initial flush of intense lovemaking is all about stimulating oxytocin. This is the bonding hormone and we are hardwired for this response, because one of the things that oxytocin helps us to do is to establish the trust that bonds us to our mate.

Now I do realise that when a couple have been together for a while, this exciting initial hot horniness tends to lessen (lucky you if not). We get used to each other, and the sureness of our pairing is embedded in a knowing, a trust. This is a natural part of the process of bonding. When couples have established a sureness in their pairing, it is no longer necessary to constantly stimulate the oxytocin – and yet the oxytocin response is a vital component for the conception cascades.

So here are 6 very simple ways we can stimulate the oxytocin response. They feel really great, and you can easily gee up your partner's desires by just doing this:

- Hand-holding
- Looking into each other's eyes
- Stroking – anywhere! Any skin to skin contact will do
- Making cooing, sensual, non-verbal noises in each other's ears
- A full-contact, head-to-toe, wrap-your-arms-around-each-other hug – just 20 seconds will stimulate the oxytocin
- *Works even better if you are naked!*

Stimulating oxytocin switches on the hormones that stimulate our reproductive responses. The more we stimulate the oxytocin response, the hornier we feel; the more we enjoy sex, the more fluently our hormones will work. It's a nice sort of win-win.

Stimulate is a key word here Team! Please swing your emphasis from trying to conceive and place the majority of your energies back into attracting and turning each other on.

Love and fear

It's simple, really: love opens, fear closes.

Try this: tilt your head to the heavens, raise your eyes and open your jaw slightly with your tongue relaxed. Now open your shoulders, lift your chest, let your arms relax, turn your palms upward, fingers extended.

Can you feel the flow of energy, the sense of connection? This is an open, hopeful, receptive place.

Now drop your head, clench your jaw, close your eyes. Let yourself hunch forward, closing your chest. Drop down heavily on your solar plexus, feel it compress, not allowing clear passage from the heart to the abdomen. Clench your fists and let that clench travel up your arms to meet the clench coming down from your jaw.

Can you feel the restriction, the closed barrier, the blocking of energies in or out?

This is a place of resistance.

As an acupuncturist I work with people's energies for a living, and I am very familiar with the feelings I am describing.

One of the most significant dilemmas for couples trying to conceive, in particular for the woman, is the subconscious battle in the psyche between the overwhelming desire to be pregnant and the fear of not becoming pregnant.

This is often reflected in body language, without any conscious awareness. Closing our heart blocks our sexual flow.

This battle between resistance and reception also affects men, often manifesting as work stress. Feeling the pressure to bring home the bacon, and to maintain being a Don-Juan-Cassanova-powerhouse of a lover can contribute to the revolving door of responsibility-driven stress.

What is common in TTC couples (women in particular) is the flipping from fear to hope, again and again, until such time as the hope begins to dwindle and the fear becomes the more commonplace stance. When this happens the body goes into a stress response.

- Hope: 'Maybe this is the month that a conception will happen!'
warring with ...
- Fear: 'Maybe I can never get pregnant!'
- 'His sperm isn't strong enough.'
- 'My endometrium is too thin.'
- 'I don't ovulate.'
- 'I don't deserve to be a mother.'
- 'It will never happen for us ...'

All of these unbidden thoughts are a kind of protection mechanism:

- *'If I leave this drop of self-doubt within me then I will not be as disappointed if it doesn't happen ...'*

This is a common misconception, for women in particular, believing that if they hold back that somehow it will hurt less if conception doesn't happen. We will take a more detailed look at the ways that you can keep an open heart and still be protected from feeling devastated – without holding back.

If we can stay in an open-hearted place, conception is much more likely.

Pregnancy is a receptive process

In the wise words of respected fertility practitioner Emma Cannon: 'pregnancy is a receptive process; it is not something we can achieve'.

If we are doing all the right things in an effort to get pregnant but within a clenched endeavour, we can close down the very processes that lead to conception.

In this book, I would like to advocate a culture of nurturing our fertility. To embrace the right foods, the right kind of rest, the right avoidance of toxic substances that inhibit our fertility, the right kind of free-flowing loving – but without the *doing-right* becoming a stress in itself.

A hugely important part of conception is the body's need to know that it has the wherewithal to conceive, to gestate (that is, to carry a foetus in the womb from conception to birth), to have the strength and power for delivery and recovery, and enough energy to parent that newborn/infant/toddler/child through all those early stages of childhood.

By applying positive habits to all the good things we are doing in respect of diet and lifestyle we automatically place ourselves into a receptive mode, affirming in our hearts and minds the willingness to receive. Preparing for a healthy pregnancy does make us more receptive.

We also need to have the patience to respect that the multiplicity of aspects that need to be in play for that conception to happen relies on the synergy of a myriad things converging simultaneously ... (whew! What a sentence) ... in other words, a dose of magic. There is naught that we can do to ensure conception, so it is important, in waiting to conceive, that we cultivate our patience.

Dare to imagine

Conception is about much, much more than a sperm fertilising an egg.

Time and time again in my practice I find I am working with couples who are deeply focused on fertilisation and implantation as the ultimate goal. Getting pregnant may be the key ambition, but it is important to recognise that the actual implantation is a mere fraction of a moment in the whole life of this person-to-be.

If we can let our horizons stretch, then we begin to embrace the full implication of what a conception is leading to. The goal is not to get pregnant, the goal is to step into parenthood.

I always ask couples to put their energy into imagining the belly getting bigger, the baby moving inside the mother, preparing for labour, writing the birth plan, thinking about the kind of birth they would like to have. To imagine that baby coming out into the light and into their lives, holding their wee infant and loving him or her wholly. Imagine that infant growing, sitting up, crawling, smiling, learning to walk and talk.

Time and time again, women in particular communicate to me that they are so deeply afraid to even begin to allow themselves to dare to imagine. It is so emotionally risky. It is emotionally wearing to actually connect to our true heart wishes.

It feels much safer and more appropriate to not imagine that parenthood, because if it doesn't happen we feel we have made ourselves safer from the disappointment. But ... by opening our hearts to the place of welcoming a child fully into our lives, we actually develop our physiological receptiveness to pregnancy. By limiting our expectations to the point of conception we limit the full extent to which our heart can open and receive.

Dare to imagine, let yourself flow into that future with that child ... before you know it, they'll be off to university.

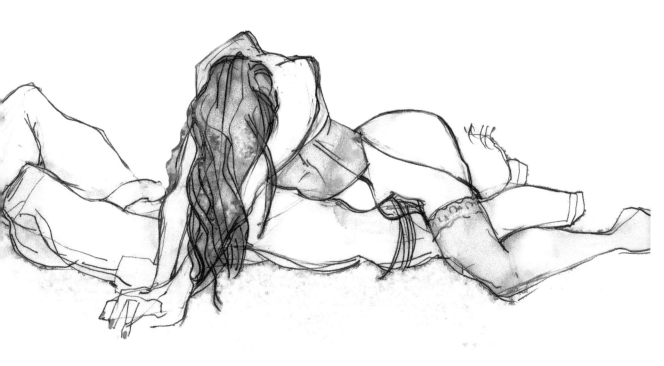

the beginning (her)

i am shot with languid
the heaviness of the feeling a lover brings
through the medium of words you are seducing me
in every cell of my body
equally in my mind, connecting on every level

your image is in my minds eye
filling me with the need to feel you
i recognise you
though we have not yet met

when i walk past a mirror, i look, and wonder – what will you see?
i am certain, you will really see me

how will you taste?
a salty yeasty freshness i imagine, with the sheen of something sea and mountain
in the slick of your sweat
i want to feel you in my mouth
the timbre of your strength, your suppleness and fluidity

i want to feel the drive of you
the thrusting push of your full self upon me
i long for your weight
to ballast me
and take me on this tempestuous journey
through territories known, unknown, forbidden and delightful
pushing to the edges i so want to go to

somehow, unbidden, you are someone that already i know
i find it strange and compelling
and for that
most completely erotic

the imagining of our touch is like electricity, running like a current beneath my
skin
firing my nerve endings with the pulsating need to feel your caress
you write the way i think
your words skate across me like breath on skin
and i am delighted by the knowing
of your gentle kindness

with you i can go to dangerous places
and you will guide me
and hold me in the difficult moments
and sigh sweet assurance in my waiting ear when i am afraid

for i am delightfully overwhelmed
by this erotic reality
that i can feel so clearly through this web-ether
this is no imagining
how have you touched me so completely?
from so far?
with no yet physical contact?

i want to kiss you and breathe my wanton self into the waiting of your power
as our lips mingle the what of who we are
i will feel the immensity of your sexuality rise to meet mine
and i want to wash in the waves of the way you will take me into pulsing joyous
fullness
riding each other in every twist and curve that we can find
exploring
gentle, soft
delicate shadows of breathy exchange
rough, fast, hard and harder
crashing into shattering particles in the fury of the need
to absorb, to be enveloped
then

slow and sweet
calm and giving
butterfly kisses of astonishment

ahh my gypsy pirate
buccaneer, soldier of fortune
licentious libertine

i am your capricious harlot, longing to be in the wanton-ness of our wanting

we have ridden through the centuries
we have been lovers before
we have found each other again

how can this be anything else?

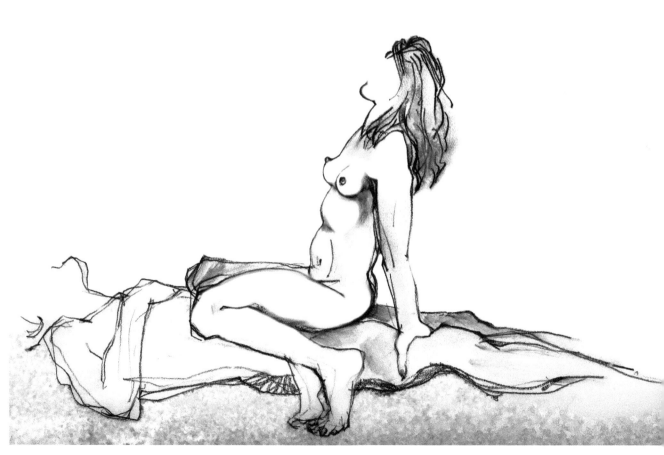

Chapter Two

Make lovin' fun – how to create a fizzy space

How often do you get in from work, hungry and tired, maybe after an extended day followed by a commute, and no sooner is your coat off than you are fixing the supper, checking the answerphone, sending an email, logging into Facebook, picking up the pieces of your non-working life? By the time you sit down to eat, maybe off your lap in front of the telly, it's gone 11 and time for bed. This constitutes a normal evening for many people.

The trouble is that it is very hard to lift your sexual energy up when it's late and you are still digesting your evening meal.

When I suggest creating a lovemaking space, what I mean is not so much about where you are making love, but more about how you make room in your day for it.

As with all the advice in this book, these are only suggestions to help stimulate you into thinking about ways that you can take the stress out of trying to conceive and put the emphasis on enjoying lovemaking. If any of the suggestions in this book feel stressful then just put it down.

This is all about feeling good and creating receptivity.

Getting the warmth back into building up the 'hot'

Many couples who are trying to conceive may have reached a place in their lovemaking whereby the sex has moved away from lovemaking for fun and tends more towards becoming a sperm delivery system. Very often the sexual politics around having sex and a whole package of inhibitions can begin to create stumbling blocks that impose on your intimacy as a couple. For many, the fun and lightness and laughter and simple joy has been pulled out of the lovemaking, and too often what is left can feel mechanistic and fraught with unexpressed fears and frustrations. Which, frankly, is not at all sexy.

The suggestions that follow are offered to remind you how much fun sex can be, to encourage you to remember the little ways in which you can fire up your sexual energy, and to explain what can happen when we focus a little more attention on seducing our lovers.

Hot Tip 1: Make love on an empty stomach!

Trying to raise our sexual energy when we have a full stomach and our body's hormones are focused on digestion is physiologically challenging. Much better to take that empty stomach into a session of wild and passionate sex, then bring your even more heightened appetite to the kitchen – post nookie.

Be aware if you need a snack to tide you through the shagging. Sometimes we can get home from work and be a bit hypoglycaemic – meaning our blood sugar is a bit low. That is usually characterised by hunger pangs, irritability, feeling a bit light-headed, and maybe a slightly paler complexion. Tide yourself over with a low GI snack (meaning foods with a low glycaemic index) rather than fast carbs such as crisps or sugary treats. Oatcakes with hummus or cheese are perfect, sustaining your energy without filling you up.

The best thing you can do is fill up on a big hot lunch in the middle of your day, so that you can come home to fabulous sex followed by a light meal like scrambled egg on toast.

Hot Tip 2: Mornings are for quickies!

Creating a Fizzy space is all about bringing the erotic back into your space together.

Isn't it great to go into work with that certain smile, knowing that you started your day with a little naughtiness? Nothing that took much time out of your getting-ready-for-work schedule, but easy to incorporate if you set the alarm 10–15 minutes earlier and seduce your lover just before (or perhaps in) the shower.

Not to mention with the help of his morning glory. Starting your day with a full-body naked hug can trigger the oxytocin that can lead to the wham-bam-thank-you-ma'am quickie ... but maybe morning sex is not your thing. There are many ways to be erotic without intercourse. Set off into your day with a memory of your lover soaping you in the shower, appreciating you, feeling you, putting a little excitement into your imagination – firing up all those desire hormones so that all day long you are waiting for the chance to have your lover more fully.

Hot Tip 3: Make seduction your priority

When you come through the door, tired from your long day and commute, rather than dropping immediately into the usual routine, focus on seducing your lover ...

It's important to try to change the energy.

A bath or shower is a great way to make that shift: a) it gets you naked, b) you wash away the cares of the day, c) soaping can be a very erotic game, and d) immersion in water refreshes your body and your energy.

Candlelight will change the ambience, bringing a sexy glow into the space. We feel more attuned and lower light levels help to create an atmosphere of intimacy and restfulness.

Music is usually going to help. Different beats for different moods can help you to shift into the kind of energy that you would like your play to take.

I know this all sounds very obvious, but these are surprisingly simple ways to really make the energetic shift that brings you into a focused lovemaking space.

Hot Tip 3a: Massage: super obvious, but so easy to forget

So often when we are carrying the tensions of our day, we can be quite bound by the way the daily grind has imposed into our muscles – not to mention our computer shoulders! Massage can be a marvellous way back into the touch that will ignite our sexuality. If the body is preoccupied with holding the tensions of our day, including any unspoken emotional TTC tensions, we can feel like a powder keg of prickly irritation.

Oil is a wonderful addition to a naked massage, especially in the flicker of candlelight. The slippery sensuality that comes from sliding and gliding your hands over your lover's body can be very erotic indeed. Start by focusing on the tensions, nourish your touch into those areas that feel tight, and perhaps allow your hands to move into an ever ascending dance of seduction. Deliberately avoiding all the obvious erogenous zones can amplify your partner's wanting. Building sexual energy is a sure-fire way to generate a delicious Fizz.

Perhaps think of adding in some aromatherapy oils. As you are massaging, please don't be thinking about the shopping list, or chatting about day to day sundries, or worse still, dwelling on a problem. Music can help you both into a space that is not about talking. This is the time to focus on your lover, for if you are enjoying touching them, it will more than amplify their response – generating a circuit of wanting between you.

Hot Tip 4: Props are a fantastic way to bring on the sexual energy

Fizz things up, whatever your wheeze may be!

Everyone is different and unique. For some, hooker heels do the trick, for others it may be a straight-laced blouse that leads to a molten core beneath. It's not uncommon for lingerie to do the trick, and I would heartily advocate taking some of the funds you are not spending on alcohol and treating yourselves to some good-quality sexy underwear. Try looking through online catalogues together to generate some Fizz.

Hot Tip 4a: You need to feel sexy

Wear something that makes you feel seductive and desirable. If you have never tried wearing erotic lingerie, start with some suspenders, stockings and heels – a cliché, perhaps, but there may be some valuable mileage in finding out if it puts you in the right mood. Heels will lengthen your legs, and suspenders and stockings will give that juxtaposition of covered and revealed flesh, not to mention that the peeling off of garments has always been an exciting game.

Hot Tip 4b: If it is making you feel silly, don't wear it

For some girls the right kind of lingerie may be bare feet, boy shorts and a tank top. What matters is what makes you feel desirable. Experiment: it's all about exploring what works for you.

Dressing up helps to shed inhibitions, and gives you licence to step into a role. It should be fun to find some baseline items in your wardrobe that can become the building blocks of an interesting costume: harlot, maiden, schoolgirl, goth chick, biker girl. Putting together an outfit is a fine way to build up your sexual excitement, as you trawl on the net, in charity shops and markets, thinking about how to surprise your lover with something unexpected.

Hot Tip 4c: Dressing up is not just for girls

Think piratical, think *The Matrix*, think gunslinger, think university don seducing a student, think *Easy Rider* biker – anything that gets you into that particular frame of mind, and then seduce the pants off her. As you are watching films or TV shows, look out for men who have a dynamic presence and let yourself flow into inhabiting that role-playing part of yourself.

Always remember that women love to be wanted, and by openly finding ways to express your desire for her, you will amplify her response, which should in turn amplify yours.

But if it makes you feel silly, don't do it. The worst that can happen is that it all falls apart and you end up in a fit of giggles together.

Hot Tip 5: Playing with props

In this Internet age there is simply nothing you cannot find, and mail order can save you any embarrassment. Shopping online may be something you choose to do together. This can be an excellent no-pressure way to introduce toys that you would like to try. Adding an adventurous level to your lovemaking can be very erotic. For those who have used toys before, shopping together might give you some hot new games to play.

Hot Tip 5a: Your house is already full of sex toys

Eh, pardon?

Well ... just look around you! Those curtain ties would work for a bit of sexy restraint, and my oh my but the kitchen drawer is filled with all kinds of interesting tools, not to mention all the vegetables in the fridge (remember the kitchen scene from *9½ Weeks*).

Sensation, sensuality, sensational ... all at the root of what playing with props can bring.

The feather duster, the ping-pong paddle, rolling any object with an interesting surface over each other's naked bodies ... any blindfolding scarf will heighten your lover's perception of touch, and not knowing what might happen next is a thrilling game to play.

You don't need to spend money to find all sorts of fabulous sex toys right under your own nose. You will never look at courgettes in quite the same way again.

Play!

Sex should be fun!

Hot Tip 6: *Erotic imagery can be very stimulating*

Thinking back to your initial romance, when you were both still in the throes of seducing each other, can you remember how you would be thinking of him/her all the time, imagining all the things you wanted to do/have done?

What I would like to do is help you back into that place, to re-kindle the sexual excitement of keen wanting.

There is a very good game that is quite easy to play: find an erotic image online, and email it to your lover. The very act of looking for images influences our sub-conscious mind, and can be an erotic way of keying up our own sexual energy.

There is a great deal of junk porn out there, with an astonishing amount of the usual silicone-enhanced, air-brushed, standardised poses of the generic porn-star-look (no offence to those who find this a sexy turn-on). And of course there is also a great deal of super kinky stuff that you may never have even imagined. Sexual proclivities are infinite – the Internet can be a big eye opener to what's out there.

As well as the run of the mill standardised-all-the-same porn, and the not so run-of-the-mill oh-my-goodness do-people-really-do-that-stuff, in between there are also a great many interesting exciting erotic images to be found. Erotic and pornographic are both different aspects of our human sexuality, and there is a sliding scale between these two aspects of sexual expression.

Everyone's turn-ons are completely unique. The things that rock our boat are ours alone. What I am advocating here is finding ways to really communicate with your lover about the things that make you feel horny.

I would like to recommend a small book by the philosopher and writer Alain de Botton, called *How to Think More about Sex* (www.theschooloflife.com/shop/how-to-think-more-about-sex/). It is an excellent discussion of what gives us our sexual proclivities, and it recognises that we all have our preferences, our kinks, the unique things that turn us on.

Sexting is a fine way to build sexual tension. Adding images can make it even more exciting, and this can be a subtle way to empower your lover with a hint of the things that thrill you, the things you'd like to try. Using images can be a doorway to opening communication between you that makes it fun and exciting to push each other's boundaries.

Some people may find that the idea of role play and dressing up makes them feel foolish and awkward. This is absolutely fine! You never need to try and inhabit something that does not feel right for you.

If you are trying to conceive, finding what makes you feel sexy will help to bring your energies back to the core of the sexual attraction between you and your lover, and help to foster that attraction into an abiding excitement. By turning your energy towards pleasing each other you will greatly enhance the Fertile Fizz.

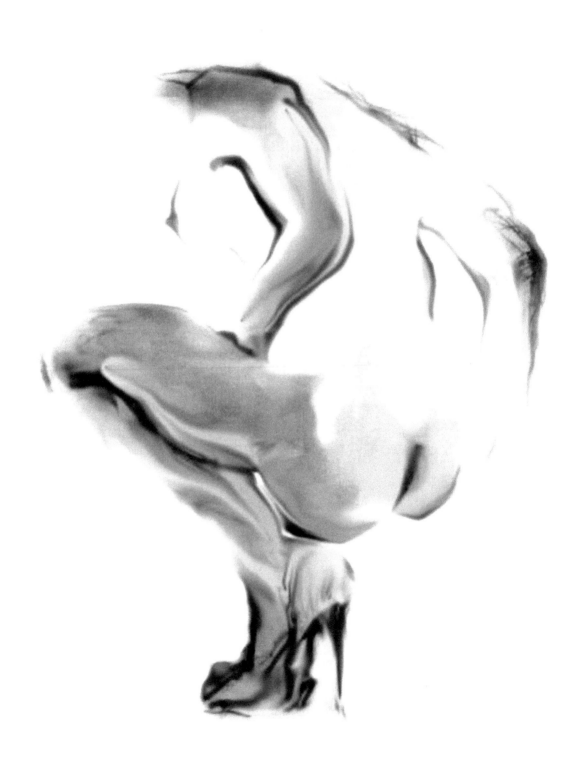

Impatience (her)

i am in a state of flamboyant impatience
though i know it is not to be helped
this gap between thee and me

a part of me sees that perhaps this is all
just words and images
never to know the knowing of your touch

a part of me is imagining my flight landing
you there to meet me
you look at my boots, your gaze rakes upward
the way you do that catches my breath and there is a lightning flash in the centre of my diaphragm
bouncing downward directly into the depths of my flower, quivering, shudder of delight
touch without touching

your gypsy hands cannot wait
i have worn suspenders, fishnets, and your greedy snaking fingers press aside the flimsy silk of
my knickers
to plunge your stamp deep inside me
and long before we reach your mountain you have felt the texture of my longing
and i feel greedy and want you inside of me in every way

so i imagine

last night i lay upon my bed
fettered
for i was imagining you looking at me
stockings and heels
cuffs and collar
the chain binding one wrist to the other
through my legs, one arm in front, the other behind
lying upon my front imagining you kneeling beside me, watching

the collar just a fraction too tight
i can only move just so
or it will press too hard
i imagine it is your gypsy fingers upon my throat

as i reach to touch my erect and straining clit
the chain cuts hard into my sex, parting my lips and sinking with bite into the flesh of me
i pull upward
driving the chain into me, the slice of the metal so hard and cold
it's fierceness driving along the shaft of my hard and lengthened hood
the very slight edge of pain a small delight

and my tip bursts forward
my finger pounces upon my button
and with slick swift circles i begin the upward spiral, climbing
a panting hot pursuit for the peak that will release me
all the while your imagined eyes watching the cuff imprint onto my writhing buttocks
seeing the chain disappeared deep into my folds
seeing the glaze of abandoned pleasure in my half open lips
the ragged upward het of my short sharp breaths
the chain driving ever harder
my lips swelling to dusky ruby red as the peak begins to rush me into the vortex

and i explode in a fiery deep stream
not the watery gush that usually i know
this is the deeper, less often experienced rush of potent hot creamy silken fluid
the so sweet cream that i want to feel you lap
this is my vanilla, from my molten core

ahh, gypsy pirate
what you are doing to me!

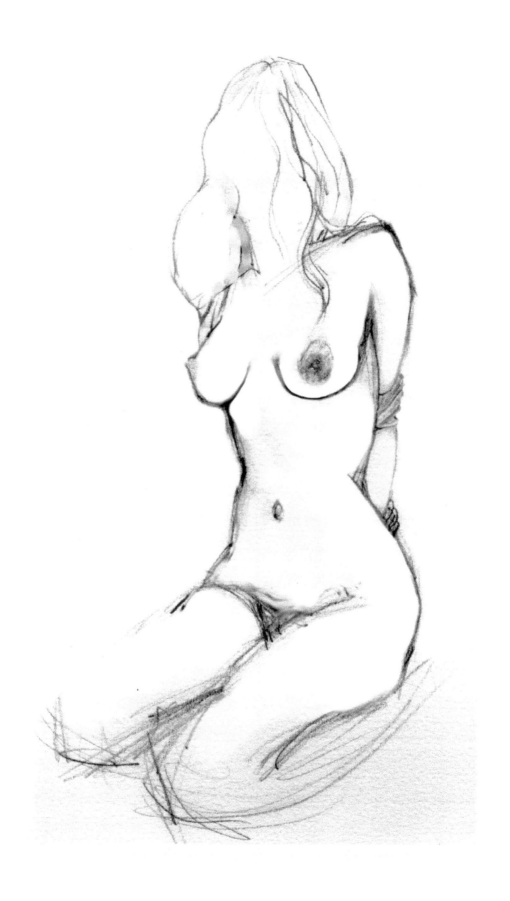

Chapter Three

Keeping the Fizz – making love all through the cycle

One of the key issues that can develop for TTC couples is that the sex becomes mechanical. The timing becomes paramount, there can be a lot of pressure around the ovulatory phase, and the joy of lovemaking can easily be overshadowed with Angst. When we are answering our desires, the flow will be there, but when a couple's sexual exchange has become a management issue, predetermined by the markers of the menstrual cycle, this can drive the sexy out of sex.

It is a common experience for men to feel that they have become a sperm factory rather than a lover. The woman doesn't intend for this to happen, but the reality of modern living, the tensions we hold to just manage our daily lives, of month after month of no conception, of watching *everyone* around you seemingly falling pregnant at the drop of a hat, of the war between hope and fear, all these factors can accumulate into the politics of sex on demand.

One of the aspects I consistently speak about to my women patients is the need to embrace the menstrual period as 'a time to love your lover'. While I acknowledge that the disappointment of seeing the bleed can lead to a blue funk that can be all-consuming, there are two ways in which you can experience that period.

First, you could fall into despair, devastated that yet again it hasn't happened, feeling undermined as a woman, wondering if you will ever know what it means to have a baby grow inside you. You can feel sheer and utter sadness, and a kind of aching loneliness, as if you are the only woman in the whole world who can't get pregnant. There may be some sense of self-blame, believing your body is insufficient for pregnancy, or, believing that if you had chosen a mate with better sperm you would not be experiencing this disappointment. (This is a very heavy-duty thought. Over 40 per cent of TTC couples have male factor issues.)

Or, second, you can choose to have that desperately sad moment and mark again the frustrations of not conceiving, and then you can choose to shift your emphasis to really paying attention to how your period is behaving, by keeping detailed charts in order to maximise your ability to conceive. (See the back of this book for how to chart your period.)

Charting can help to determine the dietary changes and support that could improve your monthly menstruation, and can help you to consider the lifestyle issues that can improve your chances of conceiving. By embracing your period, paying close attention to how it behaves, you will begin to influence how the next cycle will be.

The importance of the health of the endometrium (the inner membrane of the uterus), the development of the follicles (women begin puberty with about 400,000 follicles, each with the potential to release an egg every month), the receptiveness of the uterus, begins on day one of your cycle. By fostering an attitude to have the healthiest possible periods, you will greatly enhance your receptivity and fertility. Perhaps you will conceive in this cycle ...

Hot Tip 7: *Periods are for hand jobs and blow jobs*

As women, one of the most important things we can do during the week of the menstruation is to place the emphasis on our lover. This is a perfect time for you to think about seducing him with all the things he enjoys. Lovemaking is by no means defined by intercourse, and by giving time and attention to hand jobs and blow jobs, you will delight your partner with your acknowledgement that the sex you have isn't just about his sperm.

For men, this is a time to think about cherishing your lover, and to be mindful of her sadness, to kiss and cuddle and hold her, all those lovely oxytocin-enhancing activities that will help her to feel treasured and valued, bringing a sense of calm to the first few days of disappointment. This will help to ease your own disappointment, turning those rocky emotions into something nourishing, and by stoking up her oxytocin you will help to enhance the development of the next ovulation.

It can be all too easy to fall into the trap of feeling frustrated that she gets so upset, and failing to offer the compassion she so fundamentally needs will only enhance their sense of failure. The tendency to not cleave to each other may be especially true if your troubles with conceiving are a male factor issue, when your sense of guilt and blame may make you feel like turning away from her.

It is so important for TTC couples to keep talking. When month after month of disappointment is driving a wedge of frustration between you, finding your way to each other through gentle touch and compassion is a fine way to weather the stormy roller coaster of hope and despair.

When the ovulation is over and the bonking for sperm delivery is accomplished, for many couples this is a time to cast lovemaking aside in favour of just coping with the daily grind, relieved that the need for that sexual energy is alleviated. But it is very important to remember that once you are through the ovulatory phase and into the luteal phase (following ovulation), maintaining your love-making is an important part of keeping up the Fizz that aids conception. I bang on about oxytocin because it is such an important lead hormone in creating the receptivity that invites the body to accept and accommodate a new life.

Think of that luteal environment as an ideal hothouse for placing an embryo into a moist, fertile soil (the endometrium) and with just the right balance of light and warmth (the love you have for each other) to allow that seed to germinate and sprout. Lovemaking has the power to invest the lower abdomen with the energy to generate that light and warmth.

That is why we talk of loving as 'lighting us up', and speak of the 'warm glow' that comes with good loving; why firelight and candlelight are so enhancing to lovemaking; why loving 'sparks' us, why we talk about the 'fire' of love.

Glow is an important word here. By lovemaking, I don't just mean sex, I mean anything and everything we can do to each other to make us *glow*. This is light and warmth.

The luteal phase can be a particularly tense time, especially for the woman, more so if she is already prone to premenstrual syndrome (PMS), and I wish to advocate how much a loving touch can help to enhance receptivity through engendering a certain kind of glow. I want to remind you how much fun sex can be, and to emphasise the love in lovemaking. We can make love by just gazing into each other's eyes.

The luteal phase is a time for emphasising our connection to each other. It is amazing how a loving touch can lead from cuddling and hand-holding towards the desire to be in much fuller contact. In the same way that we understand the skin to skin contact of newborn to mother stimulates the bonding process, skin to skin contact with your lover will engender the same hormonal responses of bonding, letting the love flow.

Bonding, cementing your pledge, being in partnership, feeling ready to become parents together is a very significant aspect of the Fizz of conception. Non-sexual contact to show how much you cherish each other is a sure-fire way to fire up the Fizz.

Please remember that we need to pay attention to maintaining the Fizz throughout the whole of the cycle, not just around ovulation. Sexy loving, not just intercourse, should be an objective that underlies all your connection and contact with each other.

Timing your lovemaking – the biology of reproduction

This section is about biology. Maybe this is something you already understand, but in my practice I have had so many couples say to me: 'Why has no one ever fully explained this to us before?!'

What I want to explain here is how beautifully we are designed for conception, and to help you take the stress out of the timing of your lovemaking.

When you understand the eloquence of the biology then it is much easier to understand the reasons why it is important to be in touch with the phases of the menstrual cycle and why charting is a smart way to record the subtleties of its changing tides, in order to target the sperm in the right place at the right times. Charting is not just about timing for ovulation – charting is about understanding the rhythms of the whole cycle.

The menstrual phases

It is in incredibly helpful to chart the menstrual cycle if it is done to enhance the receptivity of the womb to maximise the ovulatory function, and it can lead to regular menstrual cycles and unproblematic periods without PMS.

The first half of the cycle is called the follicular phase, as this is the time for the development of the follicle, and the second half of the cycle is called the luteal phase, where fertilisation and implantation may occur. Once there has been an ovulation, the follicle has released the egg. At the moment of ovulation the follicle becomes the corpus luteum and will begin to produce the progesterone that elevates the temperature within the womb, generating the climate to aid implantation.

Phase 1: The menstruation

If there has not been an implantation, the hypothalamus/pituitary does not release the hCG (human chorionic gonadotropin, the hormone that causes the double line to appear on the pee test) and so the HPO – the hypothalamic-pituitary-ovarian axis – triggers the releasing hormones that cause the period to flow.

Your sadness is a given, but we need to remember that the hormones that cause the period to flow are the very hormones stimulating the next follicle that may well hold the egg that will be successfully fertilised and implanted.

From day one of the period the next cycle has already begun. The LH (luteinising hormone) and FSH (follicle-stimulating hormone) are developing the follicles, usually 4 or 5, and over the coming week the follicle with the greatest potential to release a viable egg will become the dominant one. The wonder that is oxytocin helps the LH to improve the functioning of the HPO (which stimulates and regulates the movement of the reproductive hormones). This generates the maturation of the follicle and the development of the oestrogen levels that plump up the endometrium, creating an environment that is primed to receive implantation. A loving touch is the sure-fire way to help Fizz up this preparation time.

During the menses (the monthly discharge of blood from the uterus) the cervix is open, allowing the downward tide that empties and cleanses the endometrium, making way for the next opportunity for conception.

In Chinese medicine we have an extensive toolkit that we use to streamline and improve menstrual function. As a practitioner of TCM (Traditional Chinese Medicine), I take detailed notes to record how a client's period is behaving, in order to notate the 'character' of the period. (See the back of this book for more information.) Every period is an opportunity to learn about the health of the endometrium, and the general condition of the pelvic region, for the way that the woman experiences her period is vital to understanding if there are problems that need to be resolved. For the TCM practitioner this is an opportunity to learn the ways in which we can use acupuncture and herbs to improve function, and to learn the correct dietary and lifestyle changes that might help improve your menstrual function.

In my practice I am always working with women towards the goal of having what I call a 'pretty period'. Meaning: happening monthly within a regular 26–32 day pattern, with between 3–7 days of regulated abundant easeful flow of healthy ruby-red clean blood, with some normal spotting at the beginning and/or end of the period, no clots, no pain, no associated symptoms of headache or backache, no associated emotional lability (meaning irritability, intolerance, frustration, anger, over-sensitivity, sadness or depressive feelings – very hard when you are struggling with the disappointment of yet another month without a conception). And I like to see a menstrual period with undisturbed sleep, regular appetite and regular bowel function, and no associated fatigue or lethargy.

TCM practitioners have high standards!

The prettier the period, the healthier I understand the conception environment to be. TCM practitioners also pay close attention to any PMS leading into the period, as this tells us a great deal about the health of the luteal phase.

Phase 2: Pre-ovulation

The downward tide of the menstrual flow has stopped, the follicle selection process is pulling forward the dominant follicle that will now receive all the benefit of the triggered hormones, the endometrium begins to fill with blood for the next round, and the cervix closes fully. The fluids within the womb begin to move back towards the ovaries. This is significant, for now the tide within the uterus and fallopian tubes is aiding movement all the way from the cervix towards the ovaries.

At this time the cervix begins to release a dry mucus. During this phase most women will notice a slightly dry, whitish leucorrhoea (the medical term for the mucus discharges from the cervix and vagina).

Top Tip: Wear dark knickers for the follicular phase, light knicks for the luteal phase

The whitish dry sheen of the dry mucus is much more obvious on dark panties so enables you to keep track of the signs more easily.

Dry mucus is a clear signal for you both to relax and enjoy lovemaking for its own sake, without any of the associated intensity that comes with timing for conception. So treat yourself to some nice underwear and seduce your lover.

This dry mucus has a very tight structure and dense fibres, designed to keep sperm from passing up through the cervix. The pH in the cervix is not yet hospitable to sperm, and the carbohydrate and protein complexes are not yet nourishing for them. The body needs a few days in which to move any detritus outward through the fallopian tubes, and to help cleanse and clear the tubes to best aid the passage-way for the sperm *for when the time is right*. So at this stage the cervix is a barrier, as it does not want the extra duty of clearing up any jism (sperm) from the womb.

Having a lot of fun bonking during this time is especially good for the health of the pelvic region. Sex helps the circulation of all the fluids in the pelvic region, it sends lots of blood into the muscles, and it gives the pelvic floor a great workout. In Chinese terms it enlivens the circulation, bringing health and well-being to all aspects of the cycle – and for a man, it's great to regularly clean out the pipes! So the more he ejaculates, the better the circulations within his reproductive organs and the whole pelvic region. Regular ejaculation also ensures that the sperm are as fresh as possible.

As we move towards ovulation, the cervix begins to rise and the womb compresses, making the distance the sperms will need to swim much shorter.

(As I mentioned earlier, we are ingeniously designed!). Now the mucus begins to change from dry to wet. Dark panties will better help you to notice this shift occur. Wet mucus has a less dense structure and now sperm can more easily pass through the cervix. Wet mucus is the precursor to the stretchy mucus that indicates imminent ovulation, and there is usually about a 48-hour window of this transitional mucus.

The longer that you chart your menstrual phases and note the mucus changes, the more familiar you will become with the unique rhythms of your own cycle. Every woman is different, and the mucus changes may vary slightly with each cycle.

A larger part of the identifiable female factors for infertility often relate to ovulatory dysfunction. Many women find they have an irregular cycle, a regularly overlong cycle, or a cycle that is too short, and I cannot emphasise enough how important it is for these women to chart their cycle, rigorously, using both LH testing and recording the behaviour of the mucus in order to track their ovulation as closely as possible.

What is important to remember in the process outlined above is that you *are* ovulating, and by tracking the signs you can maximise the days when you are most fertile.

Some women cannot easily see their mucus, and not every woman will have mucus that discharges from the cervix all the way to the outer labia. Please don't let this be a cause of stress. There are two simple ways to check your mucus. Drop into a squat and insert your middle finger (it's the longest) and gently swipe your cervix to pick up the mucus on your fingertip. (Touch the tip of your nose – this is what your cervix feels like.) Pinch the mucus between your thumb and middle finger. Dry mucus will not stretch between the fingers, wet mucus will stretch about a centimetre before breaking, and 'spinnbarkeit' mucus will stretch from 2 up to 10 cm.

The other method is to have a bath in the morning, gently fill your vagina with water and then squirt it back out. Any mucus will be in the water. The hard part is picking it up and draining off the excess water, then you can pinch it between your fingers to see what stage it is at.

The wet (transitional) mucus has a more watery than dry consistency, but is still mucusy, and can easily be seen in the bathwater.

When we see this transition to wet mucus we know we are approaching the optimum time for conception.

The ovulatory phase

'Spinn' mucus (from *spinnbarkeit*, the German word meaning 'spinability' – able to be drawn out into a strand) is the stretchy 'egg-white' mucus that is the 12–48 hour precursor to ovulation. Spinn mucus has a very wide, open-fibre structure that is very receptive to the sperm, with the best possible pH balance, nicely alkaline to accept and embrace the sperm, with a nourishing balance of carbohydrates and proteins to fuel and feed them, bringing them strength and endurance for the long swim ahead.

Not only is spinn mucus designed to care for the sperm, but it also helps the sperm to pass freely up and through the cervix (the hardest part of their journey) and actually accelerates them, allowing the maximum amount to pass into the womb. Genius design. While you are on your spinn, tilting the hips to pool the sperm against the cervix is really worthwhile. More on this later.

Biologically, the LH surge and the spinn mucus should roughly coincide, as the LH surge is also a 12–48 hour precursor to ovulation. Now, the reason that we want to be making love over these particular days is another fine aspect of the design. Sperm live for about 72 hours, and it can take about 12–48 hours for them to swim the length of the womb and fallopian tube (half will go the wrong way!). We are designed to bring the sperm down to the far end of the fallopian tube to coincide with when the follicle is releasing the egg.

The ovulatory phase is about 3–4 days, during which the egg will be released. We want to see the maximum number of healthy sperm, as it is the strongest swimmers who make it this far, to be ready and waiting to greet the egg as it is ovulated from the follicle.

The sperm work as a team, battering against the shell of the egg to soften it until one lucky bugger gets through, and at this point all the other sperm will then drop away, and the fertilised egg is now able to begin its cell division in peace.

And then guess what happens ... as soon as the ovulation occurs there is *another* tide change. The directional flow of the fluids within the fallopian tubes reverses, and flows back towards the uterus. Poetic!

There is a tremendous advantage to having sperm meet egg at the ovarian end of the tube. If there is a fertilisation, as the tide gently manoeuvres the embryo back through the fallopian tube, usually a 3–5 day journey, the embryo has time to progress through its early stages of development, from zygote to morula to blastocyst. By the time the embryo reaches blastocyst stage, there is a strong protective outer shell that has sprouted little cilia, minuscule tiny hair-like protuberances on its outer surface. This will give the embryo an advantage as it tumbles down the lining of the endometrium looking for an implantation site, giving it the capacity to grip into the wall of the uterus.

This, ladies and gentlemen, is the nuts and bolts of our ovulatory biology's textbook design. There are all kinds of variances, but this is the general outline of how we are designed to conceive.

So the most important information for you to take away from the above outline is that whatever the BBT (basal body temperature) chart has to say, the most valuable timing lies with the spinn mucus.

So girls, here's the trick. Watch your mucus changes, and as soon as you see that stretchy tell-tale sign, text your lover with some very seductive messages, get home early from work, pull out the lingerie or outfit that makes you feel especially horny, light a few candles, select music of choice, and when he walks through that door, uncork that champagne and get Fizzing!

The luteal phase – post ovulation (phase 3) and premenstrual (phase 4)

I have already mentioned the importance of keeping the loving glow throughout the luteal phase. This is the hothouse time of the cycle when the womb becomes a potential incubator. We want to gently stoke our oxytocin throughout this time, to help the body create a receptive environment.

As ovulation occurs, the tide changes back towards the uterus, the cervix drops back down and closes, the spinn mucus stops, and we shift into the luteal mucus. This is a much thicker mucus often described by medical professionals as 'crumbly' or 'cheesy'. Because of the elevated temperature of the womb during the luteal phase, the mucus is literally baked into this thicker consistency.

Lovemaking during the luteal phase is healthful for the uterine environment. Sex is great for the body's ebb and flow, and especially for the circulations in the whole of the lower abdomen, causing the fluids to rock and roll, whizzing blood through the muscles, generating movement and circulation, bringing lightness and energy into the whole region.

Sex is a great antidote to having a desk job!

Good sex should give us that same feeling we get from a good workout, that glowing freshness from having our heart pump harder, our muscles stretching and exerting, a sense of re-oxygenation.

The luteal phase is a fine time for all kinds of lovemaking. Intuition is the best guide, so your own desires will take you into the zone that is most appealing for you. Although really adventurous upside-down inside-out lovemaking is best attempted while on your dry mucus in phase 2, there is no need to be overly cautious in the luteal phase, unless your medical history suggests otherwise. If you are concerned do please find a qualified practitioner who can advise you according to your particular circumstances. The more you focus your energies into making each other feel good, the more you nourish the Fizz, the better the body will respond. If you are really turned on, flooding in oxytocin, a toe-curling orgasm can only help! So fizz it up! However, any activity that might cause you pain, or vigorous sexual activity that you are not turned on for, will *not* be helpful.

Are you catching my drift? Fun without fear, feeling good for its own sake, unpressurised, relaxed, open-hearted lovemaking is the way to gee up the hormones that will aid conception.

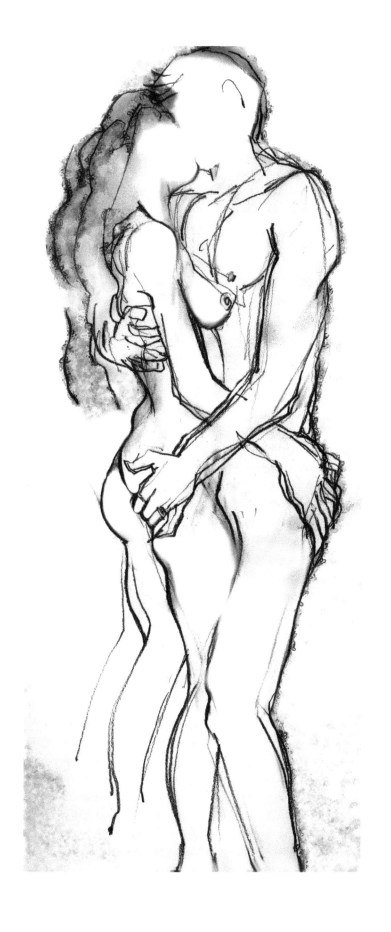

hunger (him)

I shall pull you close
as lover should
and bind you to me
with strong arms, willing mouth

the first
of a thousand slow burning kisses
seduced by the wanton look in your eye
enticed by your smile
lost in the allure of sensuality
desperate to ravage
barely able to hold self in check

I will pause and absorb every detail of you
let you wash over and into me
perhaps we will tarry and tease over a richly filled plate of food
biting succulent fruits and indulging in fiery hot spicy delight
devouring each other as we sate another hunger
sticky sauces
steaming sweets ...
each to pass lips
morsels to feed the other's appetite

or
to press you against the wall
in your finery
the door to your threshold
unhinged
swinging in the gust
of this licentious unexpected mistral of erotic winds

I pin you to the wall
to thrust urgently into soft yielding flesh
ripping asunder silk and lace
fingers entering
with the grace of a greeting
whirlpool of overwhelming desires
needs I must fulfil

hunger for you

to gorge (her)

more than anything
i want to feel your gypsy fingers enter me
with all the proprietorship you dare to feel
i want to know the fierceness of you
to feel taken
and held pinioned in your arms
willing harlot to your bidding

i will gladly gorge with parted lips
as your fingers twine their hold on me
i long for the sense of your fullness in my mouth
i want to taste you
to lick the sweat from your lip
to lick and nip your tip
sweet droplet of desire
mine to savour
to nibble, bite, tug, nestle and burrow
finding your softest hollows and breathing my hot longing into those hidden places

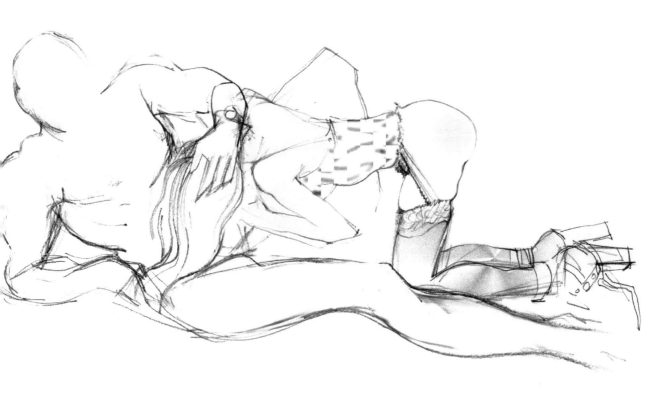

relinquishment (him)

I will tickle you with my delicacy
and challenge you with my strength
match you with my power
and writhe with you to heights
that spiral into gentle embrace
breathe with me
life's song

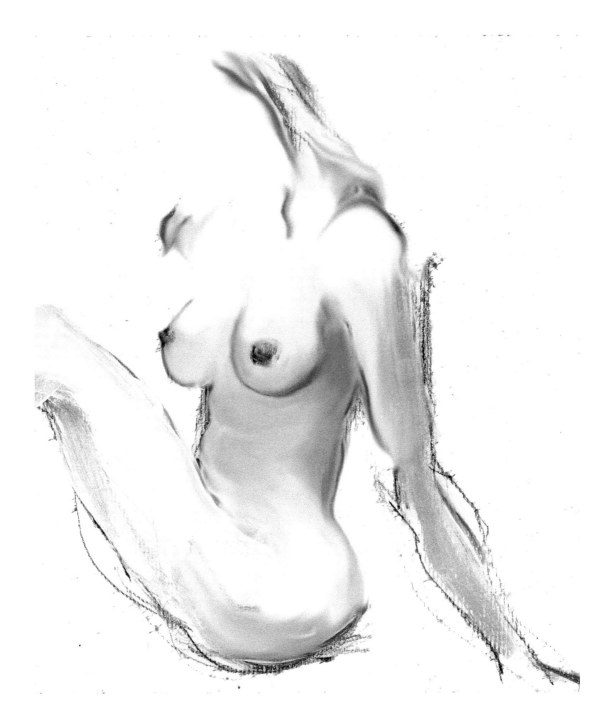

Chapter Four

Keeping charting sexy

Temperature charting. Groan.

Most people have a significant misconception about charting. For many years it has been perceived as a means simply to determine the time of ovulation, thus helping to time the lovemaking.

It fell out of favour with the Western fertility community about 10 years ago, as it was generating more stress than was helpful. For many couples it put too strong an emphasis on just that one moment of ovulation, giving rise to unnecessary tensions.

Not only that, but the charting was mostly being used incorrectly so that the timing was as much as 12–48 or even 72 hours too late. On the whole people were watching for the temperature spike, when in fact the temperature should drop just before the LH surge, at which point we should see the stretchy mucus, the key indicator for optimum shagging.

This book is all about de-stressing, so it may seem odd that I am advocating a method that the majority of fertility practitioners feel is unhelpful and indeed, stressful.

As a Chinese medicine practitioner, I find that detailed charting is an exemplary way to determine the overall behaviour of the menstrual cycle throughout all 4 phases, rather than just determining ovulation. This is particularly helpful when the fertility issue is due to female factors. Charting the *whole* cycle is a beneficial way to determine how to improve the ovulatory function overall.

So how do you use such a clinically orientated method to Fizz up your lovemaking?

You can incorporate charting into your daily routine in a way that is simple and non-intrusive, that will help you to best organise your lovemaking without needing to 'time' your sexual encounters. It can bring you the ease of knowing when you are in the fertilisation zone, and give you the freedom to express your sexual selves in the moments that best facilitate those sperm and eggs to do their thing.

Top tips for easy charting

There are now many apps available to keep your temperature charted in a very simple way, using your phone or tablet.

I usually recommend the website *www.babymad.com* to my UK patients, as they have BBT thermometers and LH test strips for a very reasonable price, 'cheap as chips' as the saying goes. Be sure to get the sort of thermometer that beeps, it tells you when the temperature reading has been successfully taken, and will hold the most recent recording until the next use.

You must take your temperature *before* you stand up in the morning. The basal body temperature (BBT) is the core temperature within your organs. As soon as you stand up you move the blood to the peripheries which will then alter the BBT. Please jam the thermometer in your mouth, wait for the beep, and *then* get up for that morning pee.

You can leave the temperature safely stored in the thermometer, but I like to suggest that you keep a jotter pad by the bed, and then note down the date, time and temperature, to be transposed into your handwritten chart or on your phone/tablet app later. This will significantly take the stress out of the charting, as you won't have to fiddle around with dots and graphs before you've had that morning cuppa.

In addition to keeping the graph of your temperature, you can also use your chart to record in detail the character of how your period behaves, and your mucus changes, along with the days when you make love. It is helpful to mark in any significant stresses, late nights, difficult emotional days, and to track your PMS and period symptoms.

Your BBT chart should act as much more than a temperature record. It should become a really useful diary to help you understand your cycle, to help you develop a strong sense of your body's fluctuations, and to learn how those fluctuations affect your libido.

It is important to take your temperature at the same time every day. This is key if you're experiencing menstrual irregularities, or if you have been given a diagnosis of unexplained infertility. Sometimes seeing the overall pattern of the menstrual cycle rhythms will suggest where the issue may lie and help guide you to a good treatment plan. BBT is a foundation tool in the Chinese medicine approach to optimising the behaviour of the cycle, in each of its phases, and to improve to the receptivity of the uterus and in helping to bring on a more effective ovulatory function.

I always suggest choosing the same time each day to take your temperature, but when it comes to weekends it's important to be able to wake naturally if you can. For every half hour ahead of the usual time you take your temperature, you adjust the temperature by 1/10th of a degree. So if your usual time is 7 a.m., if you sleep in until 9 a.m. you count the half hours between: 7.30, 8, 8.30, 9 = 4/10ths. If you take your temperature earlier than your usual time, say at 5.30 a.m., then you need to count down in half hours: 6.30, 6, 5.30 = 3/10ths. (Check the back of the book for a more detailed explanation of how to make this adjustment.)

Mark the recorded temperature at the time you have taken it, along with the adjusted temperature as well. If your cycle is irregular please remember the importance of accurate recording. Should you easily wake to an alarm and still be able to fall back into that second sleep, then record at your usual time. If once you are awake you stay awake, then no alarm please, wake naturally. Rest is far more important than worrying about weekend charting. Just be sure to mark in the adjusted temperatures as accurately as possible.

Charting is a very useful way of learning about your own cycle, but if it is becoming stressful or irritating, then feel free to put it down.

The path of least resistance is our motto here, and I am all for **whatever works** to make your connection to your fertility something which is nourishing and brings you peace of mind – and no extra stress!

Use the chart to know when is the ideal time to bring out the fabulous lingerie, to crack that chilled bottle of bubbly, and to Fizz your partner into a delightful oxytocin-loaded shag-fest.

Remember, the endocrine of attraction *is* the endocrine of conception. Attraction will always help to make the best babies.

Total Attraction

We get pregnant with our whole body, with our whole being, body, mind and soul, not just the gynaecological part of our physiology. The whole of the maternal body is involved in the pregnancy, the whole of his sexuality is involved in the process of conception.

The health and well-being of our total selves, both male and female, informs the health of the pregnancy and we must take care of all the aspects of our well-being in order to become parents. I always like to remind people that pregnancy is just as much of a digestive process as a gynaecological process.

The conception is primarily managed through the gynae, but the pregnancy is primarily managed through the digestion. The mother is managing all the nutritional delivery to the foetus – air, fluid and food energy – and the foetal waste disposal function as well.

'Eating for two' is not an empty saying, but it would be far more accurate to call it 'digesting for two'.

More on this very important relationship later.

Pregnancy is something that is engendered through the whole of us. Take your eye off of the Sperm & Egg ball, and put it firmly on the 'we love each other' game. Focus on what is true between you, this is what will engender and welcome the potential of a child coming into your lives. Fizz each other up, and know that all this care and attention to your sexuality is amplifying your Fertile capacities.

Tilting into after-play

Tilting the hips is no old wives' tale. The most beneficial time to do this is on your wet and most especially on your spinn mucus days, and not forgetting in the days immediately following ovulation when there is still plenty of opportunity for fertilisation.

On these mucus-friendly lovemaking days, when he has ejaculated and the sperm is now high up inside of her, the best thing to do is get a few pillows and shift her hips up into a 45-degree tilt, so that the semen is pooled against the cervix.

If you can, lie like this for 20–40 minutes – even just 5 minutes will be helpful.

Now, we all know about the idea of foreplay to tune us up into the state of sexual excitement that leads us into fully joyous penetration. What I would like to suggest is that with her nicely tilted and ensconced upon a myriad pillows, now is the time to enjoy a little after-play.

'Say what?' you say …

After-play. It's just like foreplay, but now is the moment to pleasure her *more*, to bring out all your best skills to see if you can bring her another orgasm. Or maybe you've had yours, and now is the time to focus on hers.

But why after-play, you may be wondering?

Here is an interesting fact – when a woman orgasms her cervix dips and gulps, and becomes more receptive to any waiting sperm. Girls, you know when you feel that lovely clenching deep inside? Well, that is the cervix gulping.

So with her reclined and at your mercy, why not torment her into further sexual delight that may lead her into an orgasm while all that lovely jism is pooled and waiting? What's her fancy? Now is the moment Lads, pull out your best skills to bring her up and into another wave of wanting. See if you can get that cervix gulping ...

The kind of lovemaking that will benefit you most feels natural, easy and brings you both pleasure. Follow your instincts, play within your comfort zone, all the while pushing to your edges, exploring and trying. And if stretching your boundaries is uncomfortable, then simply pull back into the place where you feel safe and good.

Top Tip 9: The recipe for good loving is – whatever works

You are a unit, you are a team. You met and you mated – co-habited, partnered, married, whatever the case may be – you chose each other and you want to procreate together.

Nobody can tell you how to float your boat. All I'm asking is that you work to find the way to float each other's boat, in whatever way that works for you.

Sex is as unique and individual as each and every one of us.

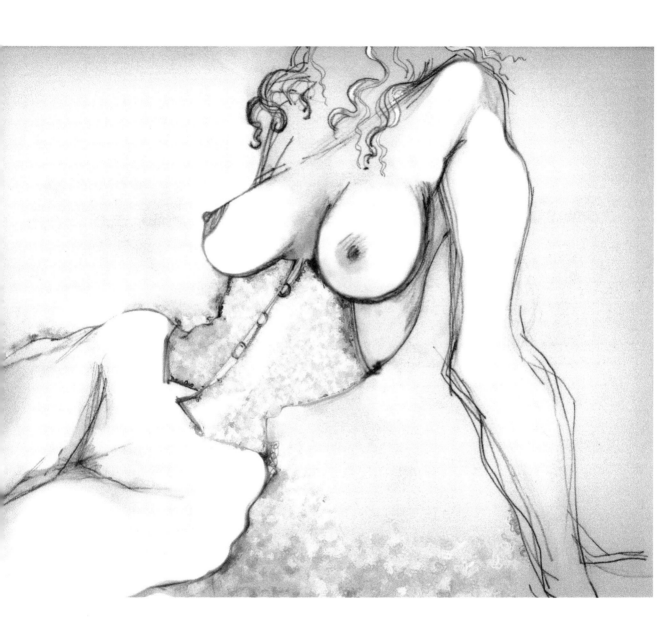

coming (her)

this is a commentary on dedication to the cause

for the sake of the way i know you will make me feel
i have sat at the computer until midnight
trawling for a flight
what a chore ...

and the train link, and the car hire
you are officially the most expensive shag i have not yet had

worth every penny
i cannot but come
whatever may unfold
i need to see you

you are my adventure
Gypsy Pirate of Benidoliege

take me to your villa and ravage me
unleash your beast
i will meet your every whim and desire
your harlot of extravagant pleasures

bind me with your passion
fetter me in your desires
and seal me with a kiss

in freedom
my libertine
i choose
to explore
with you

found (him)

watching
hazy shafts of pale light
move with infinite slowness
across a darkened room
strewn with crumpled, discarded layers

a bed
destroyed
revealing rays, touch
upon your sleeping form
painting you with the cool dawn light

you breathe
so quietly
soft breasts rise and fall
caressed by lips
longed for

so silent now the room
I watch you stir
ache deep within
rising with the dawn
I touch you

flight (him)

a butterfly
so sensual
rests
upon my fingertip
an open hand
no trap
no clenched fist
with fingered bars

but free to fly
whirl upon the air
so many flowers
so I watch
amazed
adoring every moment
that she stays

peacock butterfly
dressed
in shimmering
transforming hues
ethereal
wingtips brush
electric

infused
entranced
I soak her in
inhale
dream
exhale
art

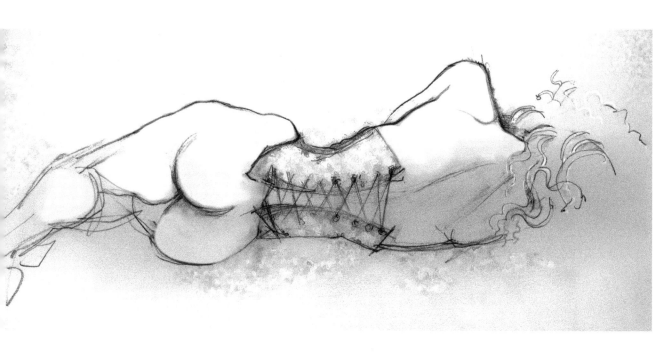

Chapter Five

Back to the chemistry of the Fizz:
understanding the autonomic nervous system

In this section I want to give you a simplified neurobiology lesson. We are going to look at the way that stress affects the body, in particular the effect it has on the endocrine (the glands that produce hormones) system. But before we go there, I want reassure you that once we finish talking about stress we will spend even longer talking about all the good things you can do to change those stress responses.

Sympathetic versus parasympathetic

Our nervous systems are a miraculous aspect of our physiology. I am not a scientist (although I am deeply tempted to do a degree in neurobiology), and as a layperson I want to guide you towards understanding the difference between sympathetic and parasympathetic.

You have all realised by now that oxytocin is the key to gee-ing up the Fizz, so let us look at what can block oxytocin.

The central nervous system (CNS) is the main controlling system of the body. Alongside that we have the autonomic nervous system (ANS), which comprises the sympathetic, the parasympathetic and the enteric nervous systems, all of which feed to the peripheral nervous system (PNS). Stay with me, I really am going to keep this simple.

Let's stay focused on the autonomic nervous system (ANS).

Parasympathetic and sympathetic are two halves of the autonomic, governed in the neurological brain. We are either in one or the other (in simplistic terms), and the body has a fluent ability to switch easily from one to the other as required. This is the system that governs all the automatic physiology that we don't have to think about in order to function: breathing, circulation, sweating (temperature control), digestion and reproduction.

The parasympathetic is a regulating system for our normal functioning. It is referred to as the 'rest and digest' system. The sympathetic system is our 'fight or flight' response and will kick in when we believe we are in danger, or when we are exposed to stress. It can also be triggered by psychological factors, and just the *anticipation* of a stress can set us into sympathetic response.

Unfortunately the psychological stresses associated with not conceiving are more than enough to trigger the sympathetic response. The difference is that rather than feeling the hyped-up adrenal rush that prepares us for fight or flight, we are instead in a state of ongoing low-grade hype, keyed-up in the expectation that there is a problem we need to deal with. When we remain in this ongoing state it is called 'chronic sympathetic'.

How the sympathetic response works

There are 3 stages to sympathetic response:

1. alarm
2. resistance
3. recovery.

When we flip into sympathetic response, alarm, the digestive and reproductive hormones shut down, the pupils dilate to sharpen our vision, and the body's blood vessels dilate, sending blood and oxygen to the muscles; the heart rate increases, and we are poised and ready to make split-second decisions that our lives may depend on.

This all sounds quite dramatic, and it is, because this is a built-in system that we are carrying from the days of the cave. Then we needed the power to determine if we had the strength and accuracy to throw our spear and kill the sabre-toothed tiger, or whether it would be better to use our speed to race back to the cave and roll the stone into place before said tiger could eat us.

All these millennia later, this physiologic system – fight or flight – is still our reflex response to a threatening situation. The simplest way to understand this is as the 'adrenal' or 'stress response'. During our stress response our energy is drawn away from digestion and reproduction, and instead is mobilised and delivered to the tissues that need them, muscles, heart and lungs – throw accurately, run fast. Adrenalin is the tool that helps this to happen, almost instantaneously.

So the way we are designed is that once we have chucked that spear, or run with all our might and hurled that stone across the cave entrance, we then pant and heave, our body sweats, we tremble, we feel cold, much like the symptoms we feel when we are in shock.

This is stage 2, the physiologic process of being in resistance. The body is relinquishing the hype of the adrenalin surge, and chemically there is a big transition going on as the system floods with the hormones, enzymes and amino acids that will offset the excess adrenalin in our system.

As that process completes, we move into the third phase of recovery and back into parasympathetic, when the digestive and reproductive systems are swinging back into play. We may feel a sense of exhaustion, having just slayed a sabre-toothed tiger, with an overriding need to be still and quiet, to pause activity while we renew our energy.

Sustained chronic sympathetic

What seems to be evolving, in our too-busy modern culture, is that many people are constantly riding a line around the second stage, resistance. This is the stage of the sympathetic response that gives us the energy for sustained responses.

The adrenocorticotropic hormones act on the adrenal cortex to secrete cortisol (often referred to as the stress hormone), and a cascade of hormones then set up the body to cope with sustained stress. This is a biologically driven mechanism designed for coping with situations like famine and disaster.

What we are seeing in our modern culture is a slightly different kettle of fish, in that our sympathetic response can be mobilised not only in response to actual physical or psychological insults – but also in *expectation* of them.

Many people do not fully switch down from their stress response, leaving them hanging in a chronic imbalance between resistance and recovery, and leading to a constant tiredness that can become exhaustion.

What we need to be aware of, in the context of fertility, is the way that a sustained stress response can have a negative effect on our digestive and reproductive systems.

Anticipating stress

There are no sabre-toothed tigers threatening us any more, but this built-in system is still the over-ride that will occur when we experience stress, or even the *anticipation* of stress.

What we are talking about here is the chronic activation of the stress response through the belief that we might not get pregnant, that our sperm/performance is not good enough, that the thought of giving birth is terrifying …

Fearful TTC thoughts that might trigger stress:
'I can't/don't ovulate.'
'My AMH is too low.'
'I'm never going to see an LH surge.'
'I don't have stretchy mucus.'
'My sperm aren't strong enough.'
'Maybe my tubes are blocked.'
'There just aren't enough sperm.'
'My womb isn't good enough.'
'Those fibroids will stop me getting pregnant.'
'I have PCOS [polycystic ovary syndrome], I'll never conceive.'
'If only I didn't have endometriosis I might be able to conceive.'
'I'm not capable of being a mother.'
'I never should have chosen him/her for my mate.'
'I'm dreading sex, what if I can't get hard?'
'I hate sex, it's so passionless.'

'I should never have had that termination. God is punishing me.'

'I feel like the only person on the planet who is incapable of conception.'

'I'm afraid of childbirth, I don't think I can do it.'

'I'll probably have one of those hideous 3-day births from hell.'

'What if I don't love my baby when it comes out?'

'My parents were awful, maybe I can't be a good parent?'

'I'm afraid of how children will change my lifestyle.'

'I see what babies do to our friends, I don't want to be one of those frazzled people.'

'I do want to be one of those frazzled people, I just don't believe it will *ever* actually happen for me.'

'Maybe I'll get pregnant, but I'll probably have a miscarriage.'

'I'm not sure I can actually be a good mother/father.'

'How can we afford children?'

'In my heart of hearts I don't want to be a working mother, but we can't afford for me to not work.'

And on and on … the thought patterns are as far-ranging and unique as each one of us.

These negative thoughts that accompany not conceiving (let's not kid ourselves, there is not a single TTC person out there who hasn't had fearful negative thoughts) generate the anticipation of stress.

Anticipating that you might never get pregnant, or, anticipating the fears around actually getting pregnant, may not trigger the flood of adrenalin and oxygen that fuels us to kill the tiger, but this is sympathetic response none the less. This will play havoc with our switches, flipping our digestive and reproductive hormone feedback loops on and off, unsettling our regular hormone cascades, interfering with our normal physiology.

Quite simply, adrenalin blocks oxytocin, the lead hormone of the conception cascade, and therefore if we are experiencing stress (that is, by an adrenal response), whether immediate or in sustained chronic sympathetic, this will reduce our ability to conceive.

But – what is stress?

It is very important for the majority of us to re-evaluate our perception of stress. For many people, working full-time with a commute is 'normal'. But long hours on the computer and the mobile phone, constant exposure to WiFi, and the plethora of electronic gadgetry in our lives, all deplete our natural fluid balances and place demands on our already burdened systems.

Add to this a diet that may be insufficient in nutrients, with toxins from additives and preservatives, colourings and stabilisers, along with a hurried approach to daily life, less than clean water, less than clean air, and you begin to see how the degradation of our nutritional input – air, food, water – begins to affects our physiological functions.

Then add to that the external daily pressures: travelling to work by public transport or car, working all day on a computer, not enough quality sleep, and then include our fears and worries, and you begin to see how this can add up to a reduced health.

When we are running on a reduced quality of input, this will inevitably affect our body's output. Modern life is full of demands. For many people, stress is so commonplace that it has become their way of life. Often people don't believe that they are stressed until they reach the point of boiling over or bursting into tears, or until they are experiencing palpitations or insomnia. When the stress manifests as a physical symptom or emotional outburst, this is when our body is telling us that it can no longer easily handle the stress – when we are in a state of being *over*-stressed.

Stress isn't always bad. In small doses, it can help you perform under pressure and motivate you to do your best (like meeting publishing deadlines!). But when you are constantly running with your adrenal response switched 'on', this will eventually take a toll on your peace of mind and the health of your body. This is one of the key reasons why stress is so endemic in our society – we spend a lot of our energy anticipating problems that keeps us looped in our stress response.

If you frequently find yourself feeling frazzled and overwhelmed, feeling overtired and under pressure, then it's time to take action to bring your nervous system back into balance. You can protect yourself by learning how to recognise the signs of stress and by taking steps to reduce its harmful effects.

Many people find themselves in a constant state of switching between sympathetic and parasympathetic. Think back to those 3 stages of the sympathetic response: alarm, resistance, recovery. What happens in the sustained state of stress is that we waver between alarm and resistance, but often do not switch down fully into recovery. This is the *switchy mechanism* I will refer to later in this book, and it can play havoc with our digestive and reproductive systems. This may go a long way to explaining what is diagnosed as IBS (irritable bowel syndrome). If you suffer from uncomfortable, fluctuating digestive symptoms, it is important to consider whether this may be stemming from sympathetic response overload.

The effects of elevated cortisol

Did you know that your adrenal glands are actually 2 glands, one inside the other?

The adrenal medulla is in the centre, and the adrenal cortex is around the outside of the medulla. The medulla is where your fight or flight mechanism is situated and it releases the catecholamines: adrenalin and noreadrenalin.

The cortex produces the corticosteroids: aldosterone helps to control your blood pressure and volume, cortisol regulates the metabolism of glucose, particularly in times of stress, and the adrenal cortex produces the sex steroids – androgens, oestrogens and progesterone.

Adrenal androgens are much less potent than testicular androgens and they are the source of androgens for females, important for libido. For males, the adrenal cortex is the source of oestrogen, important for the maturation of sperm, and may be connected to healthy male libido.

Chronic sympathetic state is often the key to why so many people experience low libido.

Cortisol is referred to as the body's stress hormone. When we are stressed our cortisol levels are elevated, blood pressure increases and our immune function is suppressed. Over time this can have significant impact on all our body's systems.

Cortisol's principal function is controlling the body's blood sugar levels and thus it plays a very significant role in regulating metabolism. This is very important in understanding the relationship between the balance of our digestive and our reproductive hormones, which we will discuss later.

When we are in a state of chronic activation of the stress response, there may be too much cortisol in the system, which may lead to an overall dysregulation of the endocrine system (meaning it buggers up those hormone cascades that I keep banging on about).

When cortisol levels remain too elevated this may develop into symptoms such as sleep disturbance, anxiety, depression, fatigue, digestive problems, tension headaches and gynaecological dysfunction. High cortisol levels over a prolonged time can cause lack of sex drive and, in women, periods can become irregular, less frequent or stop altogether. High cortisol levels will have a detrimental effect on healthy sperm production.

Chronic stress disrupts nearly every system in your body. It can raise blood pressure, suppress the immune system, increase the risk of heart attack and stroke, contribute to infertility, and speed up the ageing process. Long-term stress can even rewire the brain, leaving you more vulnerable to low moods.

Mental symptoms of stress include:

- memory problems
- difficulty or inability to concentrate
- poor judgement
- changes in behaviour
- seeing only the negative
- anxious or racing thoughts
- constant worrying

- moodiness
- irritability or short temper
- frequent crying
- anger
- agitation, inability to relax
- feeling overwhelmed
- a sense of loneliness and isolation
- depression or general unhappiness
- anxiety.

Physical symptoms of stress include:

- aches and pains
- diarrhoea or constipation
- nausea
- food cravings
- lack of appetite
- dizziness
- fainting spells
- breathlessness
- chest pain, rapid heartbeat
- cramps or muscle spasms
- sexual difficulties such as erectile dysfunction or loss of sexual desire
- frequent colds
- feeling tired
- lethargy, exhaustion
- difficulty sleeping
- sleeping too much or sleeping too little
- isolating yourself from others

- procrastinating or neglecting responsibilities
- using alcohol, cigarettes, or drugs to relax
- nervous habits (eg. nail-biting, pacing, leg-shaking)
- nervous twitches
- pins and needles
- feeling restless
- a tendency to sweat.

Please keep in mind that the signs and symptoms of stress can also be caused by other psychological and medical problems. If you're experiencing any of the warning signs of stress, it's important to see your GP. Your doctor should be able to help you determine whether or not your symptoms are stress-related.

Making this positive

One of the most important things about this book is that it is all about helping you to find a pragmatic honest way to understand how you are responding to all the factors that make up your individual circumstances, and the individual ways you each respond to the various stresses you are experiencing, in all aspects of your lives, and particularly around not conceiving.

As such, please be aware of the need to try to open this fully to the whole spectrum of thoughts and feelings, the whole spectrum of fertility factors, the whole spectrum of people's differing daily lives and circumstances, and not least, to the whole spectrum of how sexual politics can become an inhibition within a couple's relationship.

This biology lesson is to help you to recognise and understand how stress may be affecting you, and the ambition is to empower you to feel able to approach those stresses with a practical understanding of how to actually change them. It's not enough to just say (patronising voice) 'ohhhh, just be less stressed'.

Learning how to unlearn our stress response takes practice. Like yoga, you won't be doing perfect poses in the first class, you need to work with a good teacher, and to practice every day to get really good at it.

Learning to see your stress is a first step, and then learning how to shift it is the bit that takes daily practice. It won't just go away. BUT, it can change, and it is not so very hard, it just requires some diligence and perseverance.

And in the case of you being offered a prescription to focus on Fizzing up some hot horny sex, this biology lesson is to help you build a better understanding that re-kindling a path to lovely Fizzy lovemaking is a marvellous way to neutralise your stress response and switch into the parasympathetic Fizz that is the chemistry of attraction that IS the chemistry of conception.

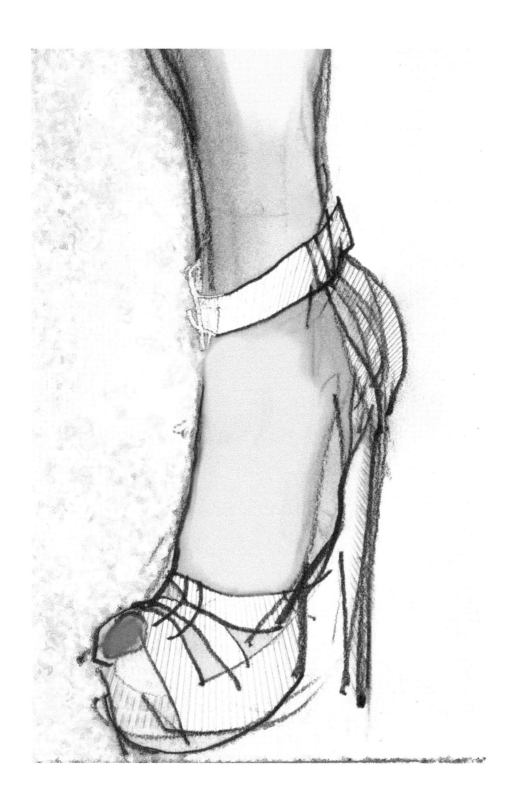

free (her)

i so desire the feeling of being ravished by your desires
i love dressing to please you
i want to feel your rising surge
as you see me
click clack
trip trap
waltz my heels
for you

i so want to feel your passion drop through your pen onto the page
a line drawing of our desires
your pen flowing the whirl of the enticement
of our attraction
the flow of your urges
finding expression in the lines of our dance

let the abandon of your passions
ignite
the stilled artist within you
open the doorway to your desires
and draw the feeling
of
just being free

i want your passion
i want your gypsy fingers
i so want the feeling of you ravishing me

i want to feel all the places you would like to take me
supplicant to the desires of your wildest imaginings
i want you to let me be the harlot of your fantasies

how lucky are we
to find each other
to dance this wildness
upon each others self

an adventure
of epic proportions
the chance to manifest
all that we ever dreamed

in kindness
with softness
gentle acknowledgement
soft sweet kisses
that say
this is fine
this is good

this is an avenue to finding ourselves
in this sweet gift of finding each other

in our having found
a match
a connection
we can enjoy all that is delightful
in the erotic fulfillment
of our deepest desires

take me to your edges
and i will plunge with you …

stalking (him)

we prowl
two tigers
wary
stalking
I admire one such as she
unsheathe your claws and trace electric on my skin
shall I hold back that first bite
pin or pinned,
will I bend her to my thrust
or rest beneath her rhythmic feline touch
such a tigress of the night

words tumble through my head

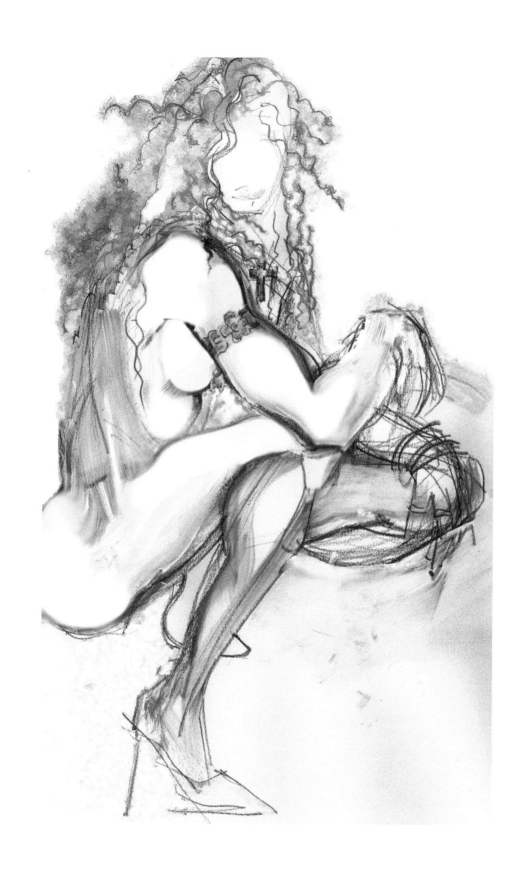

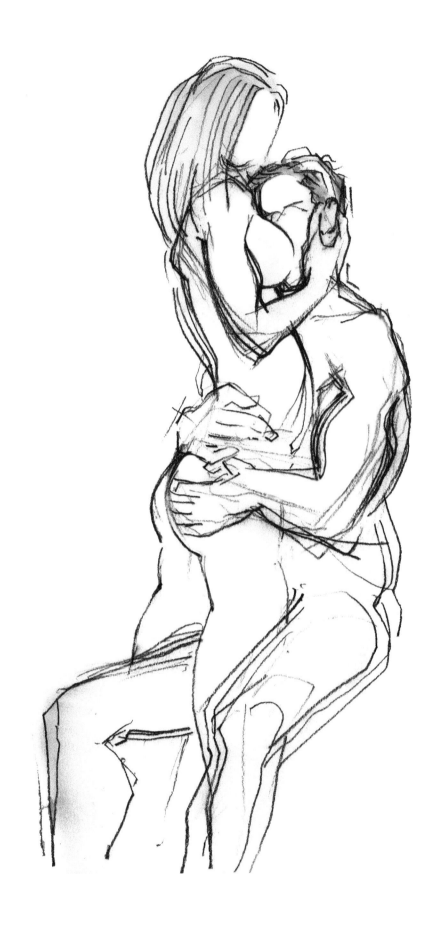

stone table (him)

infused
bathed in light
did an angel touch me
scent marked
soul touched
kindred spirit
libertine
invigorated
drained (joyfully)
stone table
cast with memories shadow
forever marked invisibly
fingers touch my tips
penetrate me
psyche altered, enriched
textures
skin
pert nipples
sucked
I drink
as you flow
cascading
over rocks of flesh
gypsy fingers
enter silk
leather
oils
morning light

pale skin
half seen faces
contorted
ecstatic
the clip of heels
gasps
smack on buttock
straps drawn tight
hips ... held firmly
you bite my lip
upwelling
thrust
inside bruised livid flesh
my soul flows into you
scents
sweat
cum
jism
lust
exhaustion
you take all
and give in equal measure
I smile and miss my lover
so I touch her with words
as she touches me
my muse
inspires

adventure (her)

ahh, my libertine
what an adventure you are

sated with gladness am i
to have known this with you

i give over to the magic inherent in this encounter
the gods have decided we must know each other
mysterious forces
insist

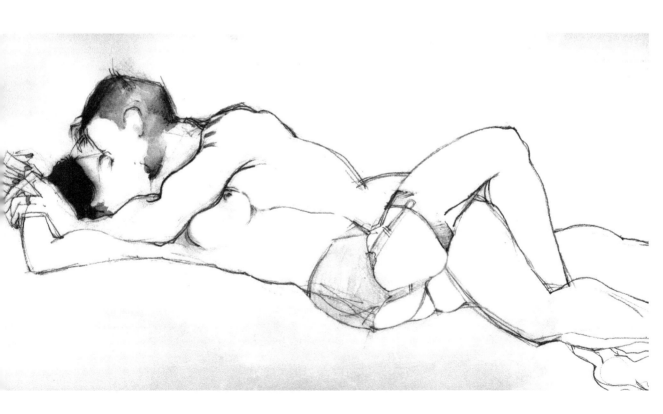

Chapter Six

Switchy stresses around conceiving / not conceiving

For women, what often commonly manifests is the switch between an ingrained fear that they may never conceive, flipping with the blind hope that this month it *will* happen – always holding a part of themselves back, fearing that they may never be one of those bumps needing a seat on the tube or bus, that they will never be the one behind that pushchair – all the while, wishing so *desperately* to be one of those mums. This constant shift between hope and despair can flip us between sympathetic and parasympathetic.

Men too may experience this roller coaster. They may feel desperate to deliver the goods, and yet the pressure to perform can have the opposite effect.

When stress hormones come into play they will block the attraction and excitement cascade that leads so easily to that sexual surge. When the sympathetic switch is on it is more difficult to get a hard on, which can then spiral into a quagmire of negative feelings.

For men, the complexities of switchy emotions are often wrapped up in a sense of responsibility, in the need to be the main hunter-gatherer at Tesco or Sainsbury's, slaying the woolly mammoth (all the while fending off sabre-toothed tigers) to bring home enough to clothe, shelter and feed their family. This is complicated by the reality of our current culture, as usually both partners need to work in order to sustain economic stability.

These stressful feelings can be hugely compounded when the issue is due to low sperm parameters (as mentioned, 40 per cent of fertility issues are male factor), and men may feel under pressure to improve their lifestyle in order to better their sperm quality.

The discipline of maintaining a good diet, and perhaps the need to lose weight (very important to fertility, for both sexes), trying to add in the right kind of exercise, maybe taking supplements or herbs, managing minimal or no drinking in an alcohol-orientated work culture (a significant issue for many professional men), are all potential stressors.

It is ironic that the very changes that may improve sperm quality and regulate the menstrual cycle may become a stress in themselves.

Finding the work/life balance between keeping the finances in good nick along with keeping yourselves in the best of health can be quite challenging. And then add feelings of resentment if those lifestyle changes are not being embraced by one's partner, or the feeling that one is being *made* to do something ... errrk, the politics! Then there is the anticipation of the stress of affording/not affording life with children that can so often be a major issue for couples.

Money matters

For men, the issues that most often influence their stress levels are commonly work/finance related: busy days, the commute factor, maybe not actually liking their job very much, or having a difficult boss/colleague. There may be fears that their income will not be sufficient, especially in the light of her need to not work while the baby is little, or concerns that a sufficiently high income will require too many long hours away, and that the commitments of the job may impact on having the time to be a hands-on dad.

Worries about money can be a *huge* detrimental factor in a couple's need and desire to conceive.

What is important to think about, in the context of the Fizz, is to ask yourselves if you are experiencing financial stress?

For many couples the great desire for children far outweighs their money worries, but I have consistently seen in my practice that the necessary financial alterations are often not seriously considered until a pregnancy actually occurs.

It is tremendously important to table these concerns, particularly as we have seen that the anticipation of a stress is more than enough to switch us into sympathetic response mode, which can be detrimental to our Fizz. When we are in sympathetic the digestive and reproductive balances are affected, and this affects men as much as women. Any fears can have a negative effect on sperm development, and can upset the menstrual cycle hormones.

And most importantly this will also affect your desire, making it harder to find the hormonal shunt for sexing it up. Ultimately, money worries can have a surprising effect on your libido.

I always encourage TTC couples to determine what you are stepping into. Don't wait until you are pregnant, do it now. Check out the maternity package where she works, if there is one, and how much entitlement does his employer offer? What is the current statutory maternity and paternity pay?

How much is he earning? Does she have savings? Is your mortgage afford-able? What budget will you need in order to make the space for her to be at home with the baby? For how long? What will childcare cost when it comes time to return to work? How will her earning power measure up against the nursery/childcare costs? Is there is some help available in the form of tax credits, depending on your income, and childcare vouchers, which are deducted at source and paid direct to childcare providers?

By drawing the full picture of your finances out, you will empower yourselves to determine where the issues lie, and to develop the strategies that will move you into a workable situation. This in itself can neutralise the stresses that financial issues may cause.

The key thing to be considering at the TTC stage is the impact the baby will have on your joint earning power. The good news is that babies don't cost much (though children certainly do!). By the time the kids get to school, they begin to get more expensive: the right clothes, shoes, school uniforms, sports clubs, outings, afterschool activities, parties, increased supermarket budgets ...

Fortunately, by this point mums are usually in a much better position to dedicate more time to work and earning power.

The answers to these questions are all as individual as we are. What I would like to encourage is that you tackle these questions here and now. By not addressing these issues, you leave yourselves vulnerable to an unbidden an-ticipation of stress. By determining what the reality of your financial picture will be, you remove the waver, those switchy-stressors that not tackling this head-on can engender.

Please let us hold all of these thoughts in the context that having children is a real joy, and that somehow it all becomes manageable. Frankly, it is so worthwhile to make the sacrifices to provide as best we can for our kids. But what we are tackling here is the recognition that for many TTC couples, not reviewing their financial circumstances with an eye to the maternity and recovery time can become an underlying fear that triggers the anticipation of stress that is so detrimental to our all-important conception Fizz.

As with all the advice in this book, I offer it in the understanding that if this resonates with you, then this is the thing to focus on, and to neutralise what may be a stressor into an issue that you are easily handling.

Workplace politics

Should you let your boss know you are trying to conceive?

This is particularly important in the context of assisted conception, although the long-term ramifications of taking your maternity leave and then returning to work is something you should be giving thought to no matter how you are approaching conception.

This is an issue that principally affects women. The glass ceiling is a reality, and for many, working their way up their career ladder has been an uphill slog already. Our workforce structures (particularly the corporate sector) are not particularly (sometimes not at all) breeding-friendly.

Lots of women feel that they will lose the respect and ground they have gained once their employer and colleagues know that they are planning a family.

Many women feel there may be prejudice as they will ultimately be causing the necessary disruptions incurred with maternity leave and the need to find maternity cover. Not to mention the unspoken thoughts as to whether or not she will come back to work, and if so will it only be part-time?

Pregnancy is not an easy issue for many employers, particularly small companies. Often they do end up footing the bill for the maternity leave and still lose the employee they have invested in. Lots of women are concerned that as soon as their boss knows they are trying to have a family that this may change their employer's attitude towards them, especially if they want more than one. Unfortunately, this may be all too true.

If you are having assisted conception there are all the issues around needing to take repeated time off work for blood tests and scans, for the collection and transfer treatments.

Then there may be the issue of starting a new job *while* you are trying to conceive. This is often a double-edged sword, as you simultaneously aim for a career advancement perhaps with the thought in the back of your mind/heart that if I do not conceive, at least I will have a good job that fully engages me, or pays particularly well – a kind of insurance policy against disappointment.

And then there are issues for self employed women as to how they can protect their work, keeping their clients happy while finding a way to take the necessary time off to be with their newborn.

It's a good thing we women have the multitasking solution-finding gene! We need to find creative ways to make our budgets and our work commitments elastic enough to accommodate our baby time.

All of these potential factors may be considered as stressors. Spending time and energy worrying if it is going to be a problem sets us up in that anticipation of stress that plays hormonal havoc with our switching mechanisms (bang-bang-bang – did anyone hear that big drum I keep hitting?).

The trick is to find the ways to neutralise these stresses. So it is really worth taking the time to evaluate if it is more stressful for you *not* to tell your boss, given that you may need to pussyfoot around (particularly with assisted conceptions), or to determine if it might be more stressful if your boss *does* know your plans, thus risking prejudice against you.

This should all be taken into consideration within the context of the current EU employment laws. There are clear guidelines to protect *pregnant* women against employment discrimination. There are also guidelines from the European Court of Justice that support women who are going through *assisted* conception. Unfortunately there is no such employment protection for those who are trying to conceive naturally.

INUK (Infertility Network UK) has a very useful factsheet about taking time off during an IVF cycle: see *http://www.infertilitynetworkuk.com/uploaded/Fact%20 Sheets/Employment%20Time%20Off%20for%20Fertility%20Treatment.pdf.*

Whether or not you choose to tell your boss is all about what works best for you in the context of what sort of employer you have. I urge you to table your thoughts with your partner. Sometimes having your employer aware of your situation can be a huge relief.

Affording IVF

For many couples, when conception just isn't happening, they may find the trip to the GP turns into a referral to the gynae unit, which turns into the referral to the fertility unit, and then before you have blinked, you suddenly find yourselves on the assisted conception road.

This recipe has many formulations. Sometimes the analysis and referral is a great reassurance, to finally feel that your situation is being examined and determined, and that there may be some answers.

For others, it may be a great shock, taking them out of the hopeful 'oh, this will happen eventually' mentality straight into the fearful 'something is wrong!' mindset. And without exception one of the first issues is the concern that this will be an unaffordable option.

As we discussed earlier, the key in all this is to be clear with yourselves as to what you are getting into, and to figure out if it is affordable for you. Meeting a stressor head on will help to diffuse it, as facing a problem will always lessen its strength and give you a better sense of control.

Thankfully, in the UK, it is often possible to have at least one cycle of IVF on the NHS. However, there is a postcode lottery in respect of the criteria for eligibility, and the parameters for who is eligible will vary from region to region. These criteria will be determined by the NHS trust that governs the area you live in. Your GP will be able to help you find out what your local criteria is, and to determine what your local referral options are.

If you live outside the UK you will need to look at the options within your locality for any state-funded support for assisted conception that may be available in your city / state / county / province.

Realistic preparation for IVF

Statistically, the reality of IVF is that most couples will conceive within 2 to 3 cycles, but this is all about nature's odds. Some couples, often the men, are very surprised to find out that IVF won't automatically make you pregnant.

Worldwide, the IVF success rate is between 20–25 per cent. I once heard an interview with Professor Robert Winston, one of the UK's respected 'grandfathers' of assisted conception, in which he suggested that the reason the IVF success rates remain so stable, even with our increasingly sophisticated scientific advancement, is because assisted conception matches nature's own odds.

He suggests that, in either natural or assisted conception, one in four to one in five (20–25 per cent) of fertilised embryos will implant and go on to become successful full-term pregnancies. This does include the statistic that up to one in seven (some say nearer five) of implanted embryos will miscarry in the first trimester, whether the conception has been by natural or assisted methods.

I do not share this with you to be discouraging. This is the *biology*, as governed by the laws of nature, and we, as mammals, are all subject to those laws. As ever, this book is all about how to understand our biological mechanisms so that we can bring our hearts and minds into harmony with our body in order to best help it do what it *can* do. This is why it is important to approach assisted conception with a very open mind, and an open heart.

When we look at the whole scale of conception from the initiation of the primordial follicle, all the way to implantation of an embryo, we are talking about a process that takes over 160 days. The IVF bit is managing just 6 weeks, forty-something days, of that whole process, just a sliver of the pie: the final aspect of the maturation of the antral follicles (more on this in chapter 14 – Folliculogenesis), and the fertilisation of the embryo.

I like to tell people this, as I consistently see couples who give the full responsibility for conception to the fertility unit, perhaps feeling that somehow this is being done *to* them rather than *for* them. Between the couple there is often a tendency to stop relating to each other in a sexual context.

The processes of IVF are all about taking the sperm and egg that YOU have (we'll talk about donors later) and making an embryo that will be implanted back in to YOU. What I wish to emphasise, in using all these capital letters, is that this is all about YOUR body and what it CAN do.

So while the chemistry of attraction is important for every couple trying to conceive naturally, it is just as vital when you are going through IVF. I'm not advocating lots of lewd behaviour while you are at the height of the stimulation phase, ovaries burgeoning, bloated and tender, feeling tanked up on the hormonal drug therapy, usually in a rather stressed-out, wound-up state – well gee, isn't hot sex just the very thing at the top of your priority list?

Not.

But I am talking about lots of oxytocin-inducing cuddles, eye contact, stroking, kissing, hand-holding, skin to skin, full-body contact hugging. Being sensual and physical and affectionate throughout an IVF cycle is a sure-fire way to help gee up that receptivity that is so important to conception. Lovemaking is not reliant on penetrative intercourse. Remember, lovemaking is something we can do without even touching each other – though for good high levels of oxytocin, there is nothing finer than a loving touch.

And frankly, once that embryo is transferred from the petri dish back into your womb, well, the Fizz of conception is really all up to you!

'Easy for you to say,' you may be thinking sarcastically. 'Who are you to suggest that, when you are not in the throes of all the tensions that an IVF brings about?'

Well, yes, from the outside it is easy to suggest this. I have helped hundreds of couples through this time, and in my experience, there is no doubt in my mind that the most significant way to help an embryo to implant is to be in our parasympathetic, loved-up oxytocin-driven mode that is so welcoming to implantation.

Surely by now I don't need to repeat how the adrenalised hormones of sympathetic are the singularly most unhelpful place to be. So though I'm not necessarily advocating regular hot sex through an IVF cycle, I am advocating all of the affectionate ways that you can be with each other, fostering the bond that is at the core of your choice to mate with each other, and nurturing your love.

Then there is surely the *worst* part of the IVF cycle, the wait between the transfer and the test: up to 2 weeks of wading through treacle, prickling on those barbed tenterhooks of doubt and fear and tension, simply utterly, soulfully *desperate* for it to work. To spend this time focusing on loving each other, rather than spending all your energy on the fear and doubt, is a much better investment. The more you can do to calm and comfort and connect with each other during an IVF, the more you will bring on that conception Fizz.

Back to affording IVF

So, just to finish those thoughts on taking the stress out of affording IVF: if you find yourselves needing to go down the assisted track, please consider the maths. It may feel like a scary task, but it is so much healthier to grasp this issue by the horns and wrestle with it. Leaving it to chance – trying to find the money cycle by cycle – can be much more stressful than just sitting down face to face with it.

I have seen some incredible things in my practice, couples re-mortgaging their home, couples' parents (!) re-mortgaging *their* homes, couples selling their assets, taking loans, even putting IVF on their credit card (at 29.5 per cent APR!).

IVF is expensive, but not insurmountable. Fortunately those stories you may hear, 'we spent £50,000 to have our precious miracle', are the exception, not the rule. The trick is to work out what *you* can afford.

When you are doing the maths, be sure to check with your IVF unit as to what their charges are, it does vary. On average, one cycle of IVF in the UK will cost between £4500 to £8000 depending on the unit, though you must be careful to look at the fine print. (The IVF itself will usually cost around £3500 to £4500, and there will be added expenses for the blood tests, scans and for drugs.) Some of the high-end IVF units (mostly in London) are much more expensive, so be sure to shop around.

In some areas there is little or simply no choice, and so before you consider a unit that is further afield you also need to weigh up the travel costs: train or petrol, accommodation, extra time off from work, and don't forget to assess the disruption to work/life balance – how much will travelling to a unit that is further away cost you in time and in commuting energy?

If you are being referred on the NHS you will not have a choice as to which unit you are assigned to, and the majority of Health Care trusts will only fund one cycle, though there are exceptions. You may be in a lucky postcode that will fund more than one cycle.

I flag this up as having only one subsidised cycle has a particular intensity attached to it, an unhelpful 'eggs all in one basket' feeling (no pun intended) rolling the dice on known odds (20–25 per cent), desperation amplified by the sense that *this has to work*!!!! Cue clenched uptight resistive tensions, goodbye chilled out parasympathetic.

All of this needs to be balanced in the reality that it may not work. Which brings us back to recognising why it is helpful to do up to 3 cycles – statistically, most couples will conceive between 2 and 3 cycles.

It is important to frame the first cycle as an opportunity to see what is what. How is the quality of the eggs? How healthy and vibrant are the sperm, are they good swimmers? Will this be an IVF or does it need to be an ICSI?

(An intracytoplasmic sperm injection in which a single sperm is injected into the centre of an egg.) How do the sperm and egg behave with each other, do they easily fertilise? How do the embryos mature? Are they developing well, or slowly?

The first IVF is an opportunity to observe so much, to learn so much. So even if it is not successful, it will bring lots of good information that can help you to determine what the next best step might be.

So the important thing is to first determine what is affordable for *you*, and then to find the ways to support your decisions in as calm and hopeful a way as possible.

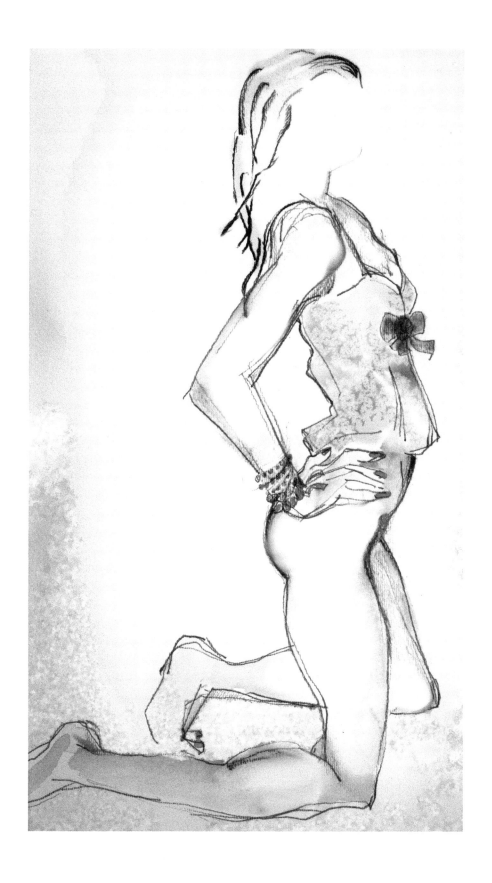

knight & maiden

my splendid lord of the night
please keep musing
i wish for you to send me reeling
in multiplicities of directions
ever spiralling in this labyrinth of desire
that we two doth make

for to be led by you
to be bedded by you
is all that i want for
and though i may be
wary and wanting
curious and fearful
willing and scared
i am
your harlot virgin
wishing to match you in unleashed glory

this
is an adventure of great magnitude
filled with challenges
that we must rise to meet
ever triumphing to higher and higher peaks together
then
delving
plunging
diving
into the plummeting depths
touching core
only to rise again in reach of new summits

prise me open with your desires
i wish to know all that you will show me
i wish to be taken into realms unimagined
i wish for you to unveil me to myself

and for you
my knight
does it please you so
to have a maiden to relieve you of your heavy armour
to undress you
to bathe you
soothing and anointing
balm upon your battened soul
do you find port here
a place to unfurl
a hearth upon which to nourish yourself
a bed upon which all your wishes must needs be met

will you let me assuage thee
and to bring you
the sweet headiness of lusts met
does my unknowing excite you
do you long to wind me into your carnal spell
does it please your head and heart
and does it fill your blade with passionate longing
to know that i am captive to your every desire

my lord knight
my libertine buccaneer pirate
my fierce and passionate lover
i am yours for the taking

as you will

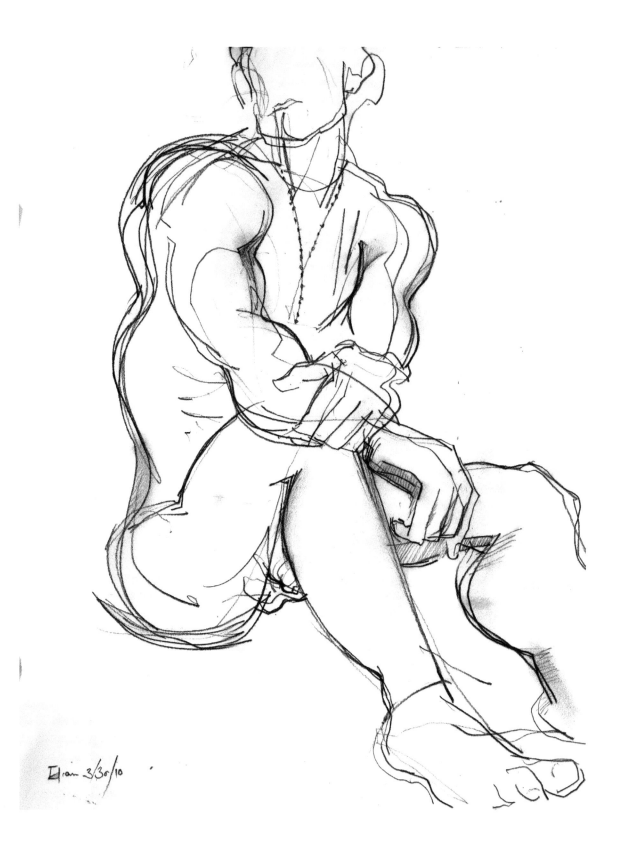

Efram 3/30/10

Chapter Seven

Dare to hope

Hopeful? *Hopeful?!?*

Jeeez Jani, are you serious? You say you understand the particular angst of how not conceiving feels, and yet you dare to suggest that it is possible to remain entirely hopeful and still stand a chance of being intact emotionally if it doesn't work!

Ah dear reader, I hear the disbelief in your voice. And so I would like to share something with you that I have shared with most of my fertility patients and with many hundreds of post-graduate students on fertility courses who have then shared it with hundreds of their patients.

And so we come to the very nub of this book, for how do we dare to allow ourselves to be hopeful, and at the same time stop ourselves from reflexing into all the switchy nonsense that plays havoc with our autonomic system?

What I would like to suggest is a fail-safe way for you to invest in your most heartfelt wishes, in the fullest extent of your hopes, to let yourselves dance in the desire to become parents.

But, but, but, I hear you splutter … I'll risk emotional meltdown! I will disintegrate with The Grief when yet again it doesn't work and we are still not pregnant!

Most people, when wishing for something they dearly hope for, tend to hold back an aspect of themselves; to keep a small portion of their heart tucked away. This is done in the expectation that if The Wish does not come true, that because they were not fully invested in their hope, they will not be utterly devastated. Most people operate with this inbuilt mechanism, as it makes us feel safe and protected from the lash of disappointment.

I hope you have already anticipated that this waver between hoping and holding back is a recipe for that switchy thing I mentioned. Think see-saw, as in children's playground. Do you remember playing that balancing game? Where you stand on top of the board, straddled across the centre, with a foot on either side? By throwing your weight from one foot to the other you could tip the see-saw back and forth.

This is an ideal analogy for what I am talking about here.

Will we be pregnant? Won't we be pregnant?

Every month you wade through the wondering of the luteal phase, pushing your emotional weight from one side of the see-saw to the other. Every IVF there is the almighty long haul of the transfer to test. The American word for a see-saw is teeter-totter. How apt.

How to hope

When you have come through the fertilisation stage, whether that be naturally through the ovulatory period, or through the transfer of an IVF, you have reached a place where the chances of fertilisation are 50/50. In other words, it will or it won't work. No matter what the statistics, whatever the impediments to conception may be, with every cycle there is always a chance that you will become pregnant.

Our human biology is a truly remarkable thing. We are mammals, and thus subject to the laws of nature, but our human consciousness sets us apart from the rest of the animal kingdom. Human biology is affected by our thoughts and feelings, both cognitive and intuitive, and this combination of thinking *and* feeling gives us our sentient awareness.

You can help your body to stay in parasympathetic, to neutralise your fears so that you may allow your physiology its fullest capacity. For we are what we think, and if we can stay open, we stand a much better chance of giving nature its chance to do what it can do.

But how?! I hear you cry.

The answer is: **True Heart Wishes**.

The trick to this is that you invest your mind in the TRUE wishes of your heart.

Some examples of true heart wishes:

'I really wish to be pregnant.'
'I wish to feel a baby growing inside me.'
'I wish to know what it means to be a mother/father.'
'I wish for my partner to become a father/mother.'
'I wish to see us raising a child together.'
'I wish to feel a baby kicking inside me.'
'I want to see my lover's face the first time he feels the baby kick with his hand.'
'I want to feel myself grow bigger and bigger, to be one of those women with a big healthy bump.'
'I wish to be one of those bumps at antenatal class, preparing for birthing.'
'I wish to see my parents' faces when I put a grandchild into their arms.'
'I wish to be one of those mums pushing a pushchair.'

And my very favourite wish:

'I wish for the child who needs me.'

I particularly love this wish. There are so many children out there who are desperate to be part of a family, and there are so many pathways to helping a child to find you. If a biological child is not to be your blessing, it is still entirely possible to keep your heart open to finding another way to become a mother, a father, a family (more later).

What is important to recognise is that all of these wishes are *open-ended*. These wishes are not dependent on *this* ovulation, on *this* IVF.

When we focus our wishes on *this* particular ovulation, *this* particular IVF, we are trying to protect ourselves from the disappointment. If the chance of fertilisation and implantation is 50/50, ergo, we will need to hold ourselves back by fully 50 per cent.

When a fertilised embryo reaches the endometrium, it will or won't implant, according to nature's laws. When fertilisation becomes an implantation, it will or won't go on to become a full-term healthy pregnancy, according to nature's laws. By understanding this, and taking out the desperation of the demand that *this has to work*, we start to free ourselves to relax into the reality of *allowing what will be*.

All too often couples limit their expectations by investing all their hopes in one attempt at conception. But by allowing yourself to be open, you will be better able to look back on a negative result and know that you truly did all that you could. This brings resilience. By daring to hope, you will increase your capacity to cope with disappointment. I know this sounds counter-intuitive, but it will give you a greater strength. Because if and when the disappointment hits, it *is* like being run down by a ten-tonne lorry …

It will be dreadful, it will be desperately sad, it will feel devastating. It will hit every part of you and slamdunk you with its awfulness, a submersion in grief that swamps you to your soul. And yet, allowing yourself to hope to become a parent will actually protect you from allowing *this* period, *this* IVF disappointment, to slay you. The disappointment may hurt you to the core, but in allowing yourself to feel the wishes of your true heart, you will protect that part of you that resides in the centre of your being.

We are what we think, and this is all about the power of positive thinking. I say that sincerely for I have studied the effect that our emotions have upon our endocrine responses, and there is no doubt that the way we think does most definitely affect the way our bodies behave. There are scientifically quantifiable physiological reactions that occur when we go into our stress responses.

Are you still with me? When we hold ourselves back, when we limit ourselves by placing a condition on an outcome, we will automatically set ourselves up for switchy mechanisms to flip us into teeter-totter.

For here is the nub: when we hold ourselves back by not fully investing in our wishes to become pregnant, we automatically set ourselves up for a tendency to switch into sympathetic response mode. We allow the fears and doubts to switch off that oxytocin cascade.

I cannot promise that any of these ideas will make it any easier, but it can mean that you will learn to ride the TTC roller coaster of hope and despair with equanimity and an increased ability to cope with the trials that this journey brings.

How to cope with fear and doubt

So alongside my advice to allow yourselves into the fullness of your true heart wishes, I acknowledge that this does not mean you will be turning off your fears and doubts. Truth is, that no matter how much you focus on your true heart wishes, those fears and doubts will snake through your mind and heart with just as much regularity.

I won't be able to give you a magic bullet to make them go away, but I can offer you some suggestions to neutralise your fears and doubts and to render them incapable of playing havoc with your switching mechanisms.

The first thing to do is acknowledge THE DISAPPOINTMENT. It is real, it is absolute, if there is a period or a negative test it will most definitely have the capacity to crush you with its soul destroying force. It won't just go away with the alleviating power of positive thought (although if you can do that, I suggest a career change to inspirational touring lecturer).

I suggest that you fully acknowledge with each cycle the reality of The Disappointment as part of the potential picture. Take a blank piece of paper and write down these words, THE DISAPPOINTMENT, perhaps with a big thick black marker. Make it bold, make it real, let yourself come face to face with it.

Next, fold it up and put it into an envelope and seal it. Now stick it on a bookshelf, or in a drawer, somewhere where you needn't see it, but you know that it is there. File it in any way that works for you.

In doing this you take a very important step in the process of neutralising this great fear. You are fully acknowledging it, yet at the same time you are placing it away from you, out of sight. This can be a metaphorical process. The important thing is to externalise it, to make it real, and allow that it will be there.

If there is a negative test, The Disappointment will come crashing in on you of its own accord. The difference here is that you are fully acknowledging it. In the process of managing it you will go a long way to mitigating how it can affect you with its ability to be overwhelming.

In facing a fear you will disempower it. It will still hurt, but it will not wound you in quite the same way. When we avoid our fears they have a much greater power to broadside us with their velocity. When we are girded, we have a greater strength to withstand the onslaught. Much better to go into battle with a broadsword and shield than to try and face our foe unarmed.

But this is only part of the process. Most people have the idea that somehow positive thinking means you only think positive thoughts, that you will not have negative thoughts any more. Obviously, this is complete bollocks. Of course you will have all sorts of negative thoughts, and then probably end up with your knickers in a twist believing that you are not getting pregnant because of your worries. This leads to frustration and is a sure-fire recipe for switchy.

So here is a third way to neutralise those fears and doubts. It's not rocket science and it's not a magic spell. It's as simple as this: whenever you have a negative thought, counterbalance it with a positive one.

This does take practice, for it is about developing greater self-awareness. Whenever you hear yourself thinking a doubtful or fearful or negative thought, simply counter it with a true heart wish. You can make this even more powerful by placing a hand on your heart and the other on your womb, and simply reinforce your happy wishes for your desire to have a baby (remembering of course, that these are open-ended wishes, not reliant on this particular cycle).

We have a very beautiful teaching within the Chinese medicine classical texts: the heart opens the womb.

You know that saying, 'if you just stop thinking about it, it will happen'? Well, there is a fat margin of truth there. When we think with our mind, and rationalise and over-analyse, we can over-think ourselves into the quagmire of believing that we are just not capable of a pregnancy. But when we open our heart to our deepest wishes, we accept the potential for it to actually happen.

By breaking down these fears and doubts and putting them into smaller manageable chunks you will create a simple and effective way to stay focused in your true heart wishes, ergo better oxytocin, less adrenalin, less switching, more stable and welcoming parasympathetic receptiveness.

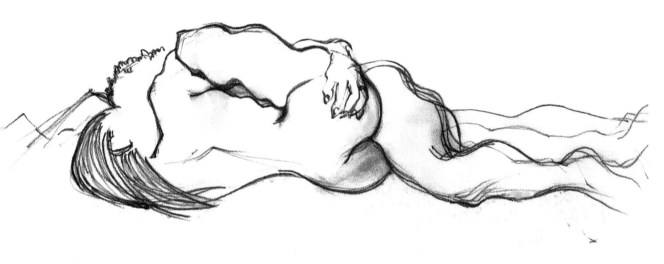

delving

the sweep of your stroking hands
delving
lustrous with oil
pearlescent shivers
as my senses atune to this new touch

feeling you feel me
finding your way
soft hets of intake breath
as the tension of the newness
thrums a wave of excitement
soft sighs of relinquishment
as my sinews loosen
allowing the penetration
of this new exploration

every shift of your body on mine
each impression of touch
causing that flowing
that quickens my senses to respond
succumbing
to that willing dance
kinetic intuition
leading the way

you stare down across my full length
torsos pressed arms extended legs held pinion
your front to my back
your weight full upon me

pressed hard yet lightness between us
a fever of sensations
synaptic symphony

delicious encompassment
feeling your force
experiencing the full strength of the length and breadth of you
pure excitement
to feel so completely encased by another
voltaic with the sparking of a shower of simultaneous connections

enfolded by another
electric with the alignment of your shaft
embraced in the crevice of my buttocks
my weight presses back against you
driving you deeper against me
feeling the twitch of your member
as it responds to my invitation

you lift onto your hands
arms locked straight
your torso raised
i slither
oiled sleek
fluid in the languor of your touch
and before you can blink
i twist
now facing you
wishing
wanting
to taste

i wrap my legs outside to in
like curling tendrils of ivy
now holding you
pinioned
hip to hip
groin to groin
the pulse of you sending me wild with longing
as without
to feel the length of you within me

i am panting
rapid breaths of suppressed wanting
needing to give expression
to all the releases your touch has engendered
all those almost touches to my intimate places
wanting wanting
needing needing
to give expression to the bursting rise of sexual flame
flickering heat pulsing up from my core
undulating snake of sensual lust

my arms writhe upward
coiling round your tensed held arms
drawing you downwards
pressing you slowly pelvis to pelvis
hip bones navel rib to rib
as your chest falls gently upon mine
the jolt as your weight finds my tumescent nipples
a keener longing yet
now thrumming through me

as the joining of parts
rises into crescendo

my hands glide
up your shoulders up your neck
caressing
twinning into curls of hair
as the gentle force of my need draws your mouth inexorably to mine
breath to breath
we touch without touching
lips quivering
each feather of sensation
sending spirals of hunger
cascading through me

reaching
with the most fiercely deliberate touch
i bring my lips to yours
that we might taste
the fullness of the build of this alchemical attraction
that has turned our bodies to pillars of pure sensation

as your lips open to mine
i am lost in the thrust and hurl
as you unleash returning wanting
drowning yourself in the welcome of my kiss
the length of your shaft bursting with a fierce pulsation
quivering with the desire to know me

the tangible throb of the kiss that we share ...

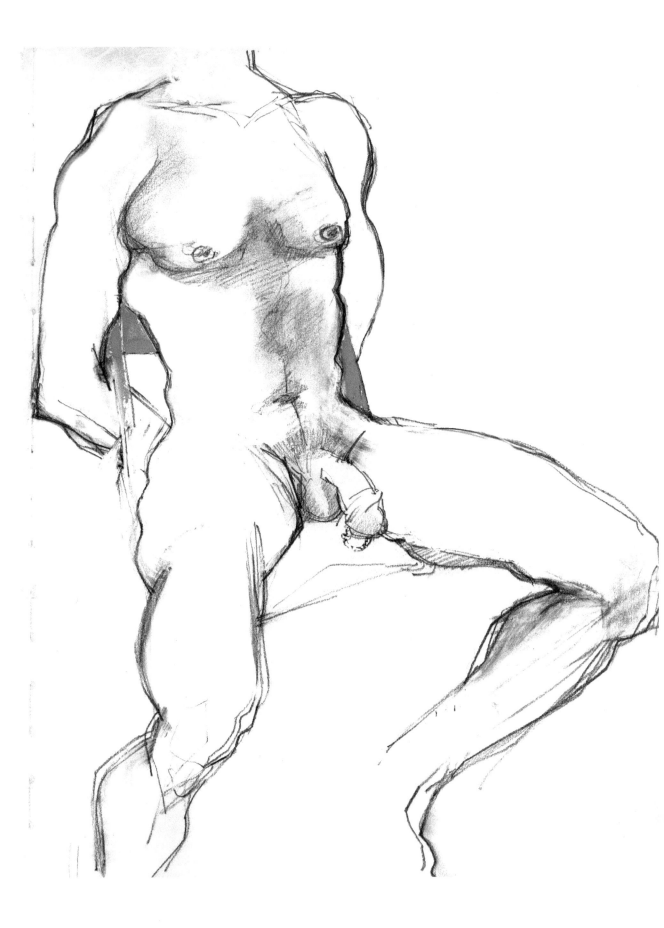

Chapter Eight

First trimester loss:
miscarriage, recurrent miscarriage and repeated IVF failures

One of the pivotal and most intense aspects of TTC is the moment of actually getting pregnant. This can carry with it abiding joy and a flash of such pure unadulterated fear it can take your breath away.

What?! you say ... but this is the longed-for hope! We're here now! We've achieved the aim! We are flooded with relief! This has actually happened! Now we can relax and stop worrying!

Unfortunately, with that initial surge of joy, the immediate proviso will leap instantaneously to mind: 'But we can't celebrate this until after the 12-week scan.'

Cue surge of fear. Of course.

Please feel reassured that this is completely normal.

Every pregnant woman since the dawn of time has been subject to this. Our miraculous modern science is not able to override the mechanisms of nature. For as long as humans have been procreating, the reality of the first trimester has always been thus.

The official statistics are that one in seven pregnancies will miscarry, though the biological reality is nearer to one in five, which includes the unreported early pregnancy losses that occur.

I do not share these statistics in order to dampen your expectation, but rather to share the reality of the physiology of early pregnancy. As discussed, a fear that is faced is a fear diffused.

Normal physiologic miscarriage

When an embryo implants in the endometrium, the body immediately switches onto the hCG-driven hormone complex. Human chorionic gonadotropin (hCG) is the hormone that instructs the pituitary/hypothalamus to facilitate the hormone sequences that will maintain the progesterone and thus begin the marvellous production of the placenta (and is also the hormone that gives you the double line of the positive test).

The placenta is an endocrine gland and will become the nutrient delivery centre for the developing embryo, eventually managing all nutritive and digestive delivery and waste extraction for the baby.

The first 6 weeks are the time when the body is making the radical (though completely normal) switch from being autonomous to becoming the host that will house the development of a whole person (No matter how many times I teach this, I am always completely astonished all over again to realise the enormity and wonder that is a pregnancy!).

During this time, the maternal body is undergoing an extraordinary, and yet completely ordinary, radical transformation. The entire physiologic emphasis is to build the placenta. The key symptom is usually a completely new sense of feeling overwhelmingly tired. This is because the body is trying to cue to the mother that horizontal is best.

We have a saying in Chinese medicine that when we are horizontal, the blood returns to the organs. All the fluids carrying all the ingredients that are building the placenta, and all the blood carrying the hormones to the uterus, are best achieved when we are horizontal, which will make space for the 'organ' construction that is now underway.

The tiredness of very early pregnancy is normal and appropriate and I always encourage you, whenever possible, to just lie down. Not so easy in the commuting/work context!

The time between 6–8 weeks may be referred to as 'the viability'. This is the time when the embryo will plumb into the placenta. In the first 6 weeks, while the placenta is forming, the embryo is simply doubling, cell by cell, proliferating at a rate of knots, tucked safely into its niche in the endometrium. Within the embryo the coding within the DNA is laying down the pathways that will become the form, to house the person who will become.

It is during this time that the connection between the placenta to the embryo connects, the umbilicus, and is ready to begin the life-sustaining exchange of fluids; literally, the lifeline. When that plumbing occurs, the maternal body is able to determine if the embryo has the potential to become a fully formed human. The pregnancy will either establish, or become non-viable.

If the embryo is not viable, then a normal physiologic miscarriage will ensue, though this will not happen until about 3–4 weeks later. When the body recognises non-viability it must first step off the hCG hormone complexes, reinstating the regular HPO (hypothalamo-pituitary-ovarian) axis, and after the 3–4 weeks of this adjustment the body will then flow into the miscarriage that is the final stage of the loss of this pregnancy.

Please hold on to the *normal physiology* of this. An embryo that arrests (there is no potential for life) at 6 weeks will be a miscarriage at 9–10 weeks, 7 weeks at 10–11 weeks, 8 weeks at 11–12 weeks. This is why we wait until 12 weeks to determine if it is a viable pregnancy. This is a completely normal aspect of pregnancy, which every woman is subject to, no matter how she may have conceived.

We live in a culture that now has the advantage of early pregnancy scans. This is more likely in the context of IVF, whereby viability scans are a usual part of the first trimester, though any pregnant woman can simply pay to gauge the progress of her pregnancy. In the olden days (a mere 25 years ago) we just had to wait and see.

So as the weeks progress, if all is viable, we then move into the 10–12 week phase, which we may see as 'the becoming'. This is when the embryo becomes a foetus. The language is appropriate for it helps us to understand the physiology of an early pregnancy loss. A miscarriage is not a baby that has died, it is an embryo that has arrested, because *it was never going to be able* to become a viable, fully functioning human person.

This is why the miscarriage statistics are what they are. These are nature's odds, the reality of the physiology of early pregnancy. Every pregnancy is subject to these laws, and we must simply defer to the wisdom of nature and its ability to ensure the perpetuation of the species on this inbuilt filtering of natural selection. It has ever been thus since the dawn of time, throughout the animal kingdom. It is always terribly sad when a pregnancy is not viable, but we must find the fortitude to concede to nature's wisdom.

Recurrent miscarriage

But what does it mean when there are repeated miscarriages?

There are many reasons why this may be happening, and it is important to discuss this with your GP and/or your gynaecologist or fertility consultant.

You will not be diagnosed with recurrent miscarriage (in the UK) until it has happened 3 consecutive times, and under NHS care there will be no investigative work until after the third miscarriage. This is due to how normal miscarriage actually is: you may easily enough have 2 non-viable embryos in a row.

It is important to establish when the embryo may be arresting. If it is repeatedly happening in week 5 then there may be immunological issues at play. The exploration of immunological issues in fertility is still at the very beginning of its scientific journey, and there is much that is not understood. One aspect that may be analysed is the woman's NK cells, the unfortunately named 'natural killer' cells. It is important to remember that the way in which these are evaluated will be different from place to place, there is much conflicting information about this online, and the treatment is still very experimental.

If you have been told that you have elevated NK cells, I would encourage you to read the article 'Natural killer cells, miscarriage, and infertility' by Moffat, Regan and Braude published in the British Medical Journal in 2004 (*www.ncbi.nlm.nih.gov/pmc/articles/PMC534451/#!po=16.6667*).

It offers some clarity about the difference between blood NK cells and uterine NK cells, and a considered approach to the analysis of NK cells.

For a clear discussion of the immunological issues in fertility, please refer to the HFEA (Human Fertilisation and Embryology Authority) website, for a balanced outline of the immunological tests available with comments on their reasoning, potential efficacy and regulation (*www.hfea.gov.uk/fertility-treatment-options-reproductive-immunology.html#1*).

When recurrent miscarriage falls between 6–8/9 weeks this may indicate that there is a chromosomal issue, a nutritional deficiency, or an undiagnosed STI (sexually transmitted infection) or GUI (genito-urinary infection).

Chromosomal testing usually needs to be done privately here in the UK and under the guidance of advice from a fertility consultant or andrologist (male fertility expert), although if you are with an NHS recurrent miscarriage clinic it may be free.

There may be a nutritive issue, meaning that the nutritive balance in either the mother or father may be subnormal in respect of their vitamin, mineral, enzyme and amino acid levels. This is why antenatal and male fertility supplements are so important.

The soils that grow our food are less nutritive than they used to be (this was first brought to the attention of both the UK and USA governments in 1934), which means that they lack some vitamins, minerals, enzymes and amino acids. Did you know that you need to eat 8 tomatoes to get the same level of nutrition that your grandmother got from eating just one? So we come back to the notion of 'you are what you eat', which is to say that the embryo that becomes a foetus that becomes a person is fundamentally influenced by the building blocks of nutrition within the mother and the father – her ovum and his sperm.

Recurrent miscarriage may also be due to an undiagnosed STI or GUI. Most people who have moved forward to the point of fertility treatment will, as standard, be tested for chlamydia, gonorrhoea, syphilus and HIV.

STIs and GUIs can present as being sub-clinical, which means that they are asymptomatic – that is to say, 'without symptoms'. If you have had recurrent miscarriage, or perhaps if you are just not conceiving, it is always worth getting tested. STI and GUI testing is important when we see low sperm parameters, and especially if the sperm test shows that there is low volume (of the seminal fluids), if there is viscosity (the fluids are too thickened) and if the morphology (that is, how the sperm are shaped) is not healthy, which usually affects motility (how they move) and may be affecting their ability to penetrate the egg.

There is an indicator that you can try at home that may help suggest if it may be helpful for him to check for sub-clinical STI or GUI. Masturbate, catch the semen in your hand, and study the colour and texture. Healthy spunk should have a slippery, clear and whitish creamy texture. If the spunk is grey or yellowish, this *may possibly* indicate a sub-clinical infection. Also check the texture. Is it thick and globby? This *may* be another indication that there may be an undisclosed STI or GUI at play.

I am a big fan of ruling things out. Much better to test than to wait, and then months down the line find there is something easily treatable that may make all the difference to a healthy conception.

There is a full spectrum of STIs and GUIs that can be tested, some on the NHS, some privately. The charity Foresight has found that 65 per cent of couples who tested for this had an undiagnosed STI or GUI. The respected nutritionist Marilyn Glenville also finds in her clinic that 65 per cent of couples tested have the same outcome.

Diet and lifestyle issues may also be part of the problem, and there is much that you can do, all from the power of your own kitchen and hearth, to improve the quality of your ovum and sperms. So whether you have had one miscarriage or three, you can ensure your diet is rich in nutrients, you can think about taking nutritional supplements, maybe Western or Chinese herbs, and you can go and get tested for STIs and GUIs.

Repeated IVF failures

Terrible word, failure. I wish it wasn't used, but this is the common parlance in medical language. It is easier to say than 'repeated IVF lack of success'. Essentially, all the same advice as above applies to repeated IVF lack of successes, and when it reaches the point of 3 failed IVFs, this is the time to apply the above advice: testing for STIs and GUIs, improving your nutritional status, talking with your consultant about chromosomal testing, and considering whether there may be an immunological issue.

Secondary infertility

One of the things I hear again and again in my practice is 'at least we have our little one, and we are so grateful for that.' Yet inside, the heart is fighting the sadness; you have had a successful pregnancy, and yet another eludes you.

The pain of secondary infertility can be just as acute as primary infertility, as the added joy in the second pregnancy is to fulfil your wish that your child may become a sister or a brother.

Often the experience of our first birth can have a profound effect on our ability to have another child. On one hand your heart is wide open to the wish to extend your family, to feel a child growing inside you again, to bring another person into your family unit, while on the other hand, there may be genuine fears. Switchy-switchy, the fear will help to block those conception hormones.

This is not uncommon. About 30–35 per cent of women in our culture have a difficult birth experience. So often I hear couples dismissing the trauma they may have experienced with the panacea of 'well, it was awful, but at least we have our gorgeous child' but that does not mean that it is not vitally important for you to work through any residual fears you have around birthing.

The psychology of trauma recovery is referred to as de-briefing. And my oh my, a traumatic birth will certainly wring out some powerful emotions. This is just as important for fathers as it is for mothers. All too often I see dads who have entirely put aside their own bad experience of a birth to ensure that their lovely wife is able to fully recover, doing their best to be the bedrock on which she can stabilise. And so too I have seen mothers who try to dismiss their birth traumas as unimportant next to the joy of holding their child, and raising their longed-for baby.

Many couples who experience a difficult birth will work through their story, telling it again and again, sequencing through the details, usually with each other. It seems that men are less likely to talk about it, whereas women are much better at sharing; often in the mother and baby groups that provide the emotional space and an open invitation to process their experience through sharing their birth story.

Nevertheless, many women feel that a difficult birth somehow means that they are less worthy as they did not have the ultimate natural birth experience. Ironically, sometimes women who have had a lovely straightforward birth feel inhibited to talk about it as they are now outside of the norm.

A caveat is required here. Intervention does not necessarily mean that it has been a bad labour. Many women do need intervention, especially for women in the 35-plus bracket, often having their first. At 35-plus it is *much* harder for the sinews to stretch, coupled with the fact that women are often working right up to 38 weeks, thus often not rested enough to have the energy required for a productive labour. This is one of the key reasons why we are seeing so many intervention labours. There is much to say on this subject, but not here and now (watch out for *Birth-fit Fizz*, the next title in this series).

Interventions can be a marvellous way to help bring your baby safely into the world. At the same time though, we must respect that our modern maternity services are badly stretched, and that many women do not always find the gentle support they need, with a sure sense of having been party to all the decisions that were made during the labour. A 'good' birth experience will give you the feeling that everything happened as it should have. A 'bad' birth experience usually leaves you with the sense that things did not happen as they should have.

Many people come away from their labour experience feeling that they were not in control of what was happening, and this is always the nub of what makes a birth experience feel 'bad'. (I could write a whole book on this subject, and in fact I am in that very process ...)

Every woman *needs* to de-brief her labour experience, even when it has been an empowering and joyful experience. We tell it again and again until we have fully processed it, having reviewed all aspects until we understand every nuance of how the labour unfolded, until we feel we have the full picture of how every detail fits into place, examining and re-examining every step and stage of the labour.

Even when labour goes extremely well, it is still physically and emotionally one of the great moments in a woman's life, hence the imperative to place this extraordinary event into our hearts and minds with complete clarity.

Unwinding a difficult previous birth

This de-briefing process is even more important when a previous labour has not gone well. I cannot count the number of times I have been with women in the final stages of a subsequent pregnancy, while they are awaiting the spontaneous onset of labour, and in the course of our talking they will burst into tears as all the fears from their previous birth experience burst out.

Often as not, what will come up is an unprocessed aspect of that other labour, usually tied up with the moment they feel they lost control of what was happening and fell subject to all the impositions that define trauma.

There is a very good website that discusses trauma in depth:
www.helpguide.org/mental/emotional_psychological_trauma.htm

An event will most likely lead to emotional or psychological trauma if:

- It happened unexpectedly
- You were unprepared for it
- You felt powerless to prevent it
- It happened repeatedly
- Someone was intentionally cruel.

Emotional and psychological symptoms of trauma:

- Shock, denial or disbelief
- Anger, irritability, mood swings
- Guilt, shame, self-blame
- Feeling sad or hopeless
- Confusion, difficulty concentrating
- Anxiety and fear
- Withdrawing from others
- Feeling disconnected or numb.

Physical symptoms of trauma:

- Insomnia or nightmares
- Being startled easily
- Racing heartbeat
- Aches and pains
- Fatigue

- Difficulty concentrating
- Edginess and agitation
- Muscle tension.

These trauma symptoms and feelings typically last from a few days to a few months, gradually fading as you process the trauma. But even when you're feeling better, you may be troubled from time to time by painful memories or emotions – especially in response to triggers such as an anniversary of the event or an image, sound, or situation that reminds you of the traumatic experience.

In just the same way that the fear of a difficult labour can inhibit or stop the onset of spontaneous labour (oh those sympathetic hormones!), trauma fears are more than enough to play switchy havoc which will significantly impact on our conception cascades. It is very important to work through your emotions around any previous birth experience and ensure that you are clear about how and why things happened the way they did.

The NHS has an excellent support system called PALS, the Patient Advice and Liaison Service (*www.nhs.uk/Service-Search/Patient-advice-and-liaison-services-(PALS)/LocationSearch/363*).

If you have had a difficult or traumatic birth experience, you can go to the PALS office of the NHS trust that your hospital, birthing unit or community midwifery service is governed by, and they will be able to read through your labour notes with you, explaining the medical terminology and the chronology of all the circumstances as they unfolded, and helping you to fully de-brief your labour as it has been recorded in your notes.

If it is appropriate or necessary for you, you may communicate with the medical staff who were involved in your labour, usually by letter, with the proviso that you will not be in direct contact.

This can be a very healing step to help you process your labour experience, and to understand why things unfolded as they did. All too often I have talked with women (over 14 years of answering the Birth Crisis Network helpline) and encouraged them to go through this process as a means of connecting to the experience and to working through just what happened and why.

It is feeling out of control that will make a bad birth experience. PALS is there to help unwind your story and understand exactly what happened, step by step. (In countries outside the UK you will need to enquire with the administration of the hospital or unit who oversaw your labour and ask to have access to your notes.)

Doing the detective work …

Secondary infertility may be a straightforward physical issue rather than an emotional one (though it is often is a combination of both). In all the same ways that we need to do the detective work in primary infertility, we need to apply the same process to secondary infertility. We cannot simply make the assumption that because there was a previous pregnancy, there will easily be a subsequent one.

It is important to review all the markers of fertility: are the HPO hormones doing what they should? Is the cycle regular? Is there a healthy ovulation? Does the menstrual bleed show us that the endometrium is healthy? A lot can change after a childbirth, especially if the labour was difficult, or the woman's recovery was compromised with emotional stress, or physical stresses such as poor diet, sleeping problems (on top of the normal disruptions inherent with newborns and infants!), too early resumption of sexual intercourse, a long slow recovery from tears or a Caesarean, or muscular skeletal problems that may be exacerbated or develop after childbirth, perhaps following heavy use of anaesthetics, particularly an epidural, which is injected into the spinal area.

If you had an epidural in your previous labour, and since that delivery you have not had a resumption of your normal levels of libido (often very hard in those early infant years!) and you have not felt a good re-connection to your sexuality, then I urge you to consider acupuncture. There is a very important meridian channel that runs up the spine, and it may be that an epidural has created an energetic block in this meridian.

As women it is very easy for us to put aside our own physical well-being to care for our new baby, and sometimes a mother may have a poor physical recovery and may end up in a state of sub-fertility. Things are working, but not working well enough for her to bear another conception. This may fall into what is deemed the 'unexplained' category.

In Chinese medicine, when a woman presents with secondary infertility, we will take a detailed history of the pregnancy, the childbirth and the recovery, asking many questions about her condition through each of these phases, and paying close attention to how she was feeling emotionally throughout.

One of the marvellous things about Chinese medicine is that it studies how all the systems that support conception and gestation are functioning. We are not just looking at the gynaecology in isolation, but looking to understand *all* of the aspects of this woman's life and experience that may be contributing to why a conception may not be happening.

I have such an enormous respect for the great body of knowledge that Chinese medicine brings to gynaecology, a 5000-year history with three and half millennia of written works. Fertility has long been a key subject in Chinese medicine, and if you are feeling that it is just not good enough to be told that you have unexplained or secondary infertility, I encourage you to explore TCM, to find the diet and lifestyle and treatment support that can enhance your fertility.

And this is not just for the girls. It is equally important to ask 'how are the sperm?' A lot can change with the pressures of working full-time through infant, baby and toddlerhood, and many men may suffer at the level of the nutritive health of their sperm. Rest is an important part of our nutrition, and how our body absorbs the nutrition from our food will depend on how well we are functioning. If the sympathetic hormones are in dominance, this will affect the digestive hormones, which will affect nutritive uptake.

So, in the same way that we view recurrent miscarriage, if a conception is not happening when you are trying for number 2 (or 3 or 4), please consider doing the detective work of determining if there may be a nutritive deficiency, do another sperm analysis, check if there may be an undiagnosed STI or GUI, or some unexplained factors due to poor recovery.

Most importantly, de-brief each other on your previous labour experience, and consider if it would be beneficial to talk with your GP, midwife or a counsellor if you feel there may be some underlying unexpressed switchy-making issues to unpick and explore.

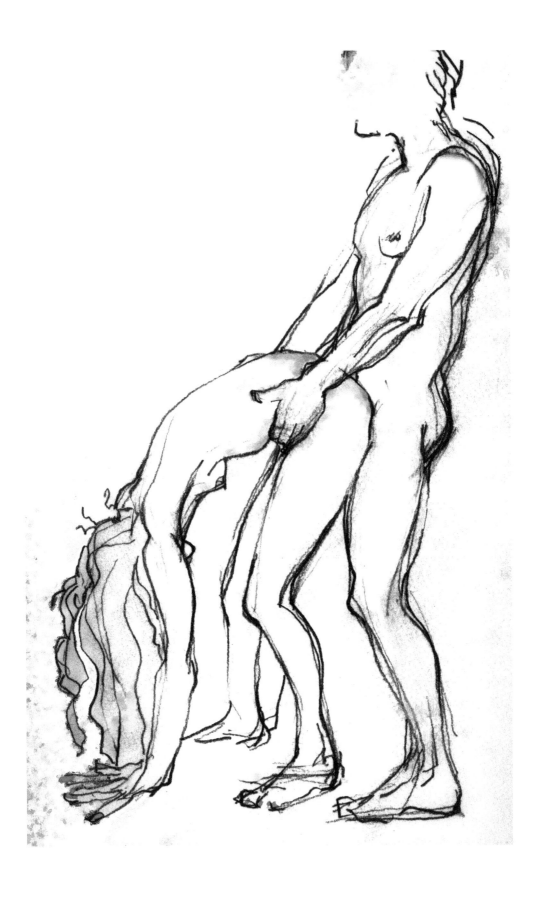

dare

if you ask me to leap
i will ask
how high
and if you ask me to dare
i will know no limits

lead me into temptation
be the one to take me on this exploration
i want you
to be the one
who will show me my depths
and take me to those edges
and push
push me hard
driving, drilling, slammingly hard
and see how i shall meet thee
in all thy most erotic desires
for what you want leads me
to the fierce edge of horny
that i so desire

i love that you have this filthy edge
i love that you know that you can take me there
i want you to feel the head of you pulsing
bursting with desire
to ram me to my hilt
with all the force that is within you

you have not yet unleashed fully
this I know
with me
always you hold back
your gentle side protecting me
but
i do want you to go there

know that
i dare

the fierce hard edge that i so crave
is yet to unfold between us

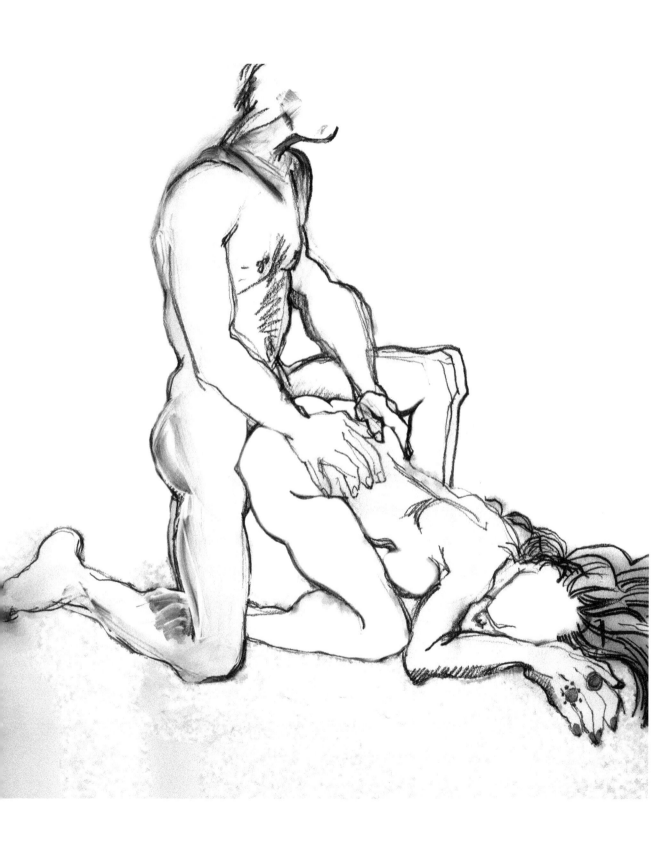

Chapter Nine

Emotional issues for men
– sexual pressure

One of the difficult factors in TTC sexual politics is the way that the pressure to conceive can affect men's perception of their own sense of worth. When a man feels that he is desired simply for the delivery of his sperm, rather than just for himself (the lover, not the sperm-deliverer), this may dampen his libido.

Often, a man's own sense of his virility may be diminished by an analysis that shows poor sperm quality. This can cut to the quick of his sense of his own ability to perpetuate another generation. This fundamental sense of 'not being good enough' can easily lead to performance anxiety.

Another major stress may be found in the effort of trying to keep up the spontaneity of charged up sexual attraction. Sex *should* be libido driven.

Very often, within the context of TTC, the libido can suffer. Perhaps he may be feeling resentful that the *only* reason that she wants to have sex is in order to get a load of sperm inside her. To not feel desired for one's own sake can be a very undermining libido-shaker.

This is often a key issue in a couple's lovemaking schedule during a cycle. The man may feel that the only time she wants to make love is when she knows she is in her fertile time. This is enormously important girls, for if there is an element of truth in this assertion (and I've worked with enough couples to know this to be very often true) then it is important to review with yourself as a woman – just what *is* it that you want from your lover?

Do you want the mutual fulfilment of your sexual desires? Do you want to lose yourself in the hedonistic pursuit of pleasure, do you want to enjoy sex for its own sake, to seek and find the satiation that comes of slaking your thirst with the lover who can match, meet and fulfil your desires?? Or do you just want to shag in the hope that this will lead to the conception you so desire?

Ultimately, does the desire to make a baby outweigh the desire you feel for each other?

Loving is the foundation to a healthy conception

On the other hand, a sperm delivery kind of sexual conjugation is holding as its uppermost goal the successful ejaculation of a sufficiency of sperm in just the right timing, into just the right environment, in order to facilitate the eventual goal of fertilisation and implantation.

Ooh-err-missus, that was a big sentence. Read it again. It's trying to encapsulate something of the zig-zag complexity of how these emotions of sexual politics can affect couples.

I urge you to consider how much these concerns may be imposing on your lovemaking. Hence my wish to inspire you back to the level of attraction and desire that is the true foundation of a healthy conception.

These politics are very undermining to a couple's pleasure, for, of course, the best loving happens when we are in a state beyond the cognitive, simply answering our desires, and losing ourselves in the shared sensations of loving exchange.

For many men the sense of pressure to deliver the sperm at just the right moment may have a negative impact, and coupled with a lack of confidence he may also struggle with getting and/or maintaining an erection, or may have problems ejaculating.

When we are locked inside our heads we will inhibit our physical response. In meditation this is referred to as the 'monkey brain', whereby we experience the hamster wheel of churning thoughts that keeps us trapped in the cognitive, rather than being sunk down into the fullness of our sexual drive. This kind of thought tangle can have a negative impact on the free flow of our desire hormones.

Lack of wood

Ouch. Something that is not often talked about in the fertility books, yet something that does affect any number of couples ... 'wood' being the porn industry's term for a firm and sustained erection. By that I mean an erection that is easily maintained from start to finish.

There may be varying degrees of erectile dysfunction (ED). Maybe he can get an erection, but cannot sustain it. Maybe it is very hard to get an erection in the first place. Maybe the erection comes and goes, waxes and wanes, subject to the vagaries of the monkey brain.

Worst of all, perhaps he cannot get an erection in the first place.

There are many reasons why a man may suffer erectile dysfunction. It is important to rule out any physical, organic reason as to why it may be difficult to get an erection – and there is a very simple way you can begin to determine whether or not erectile dysfunction may be either physical or mental/emotional in origin. *Is there a morning glory?*

Or, to give it its medical terminology, nocturnal penile tumescence (NPT). Every man *should* wake up with a stiffy, it is a sign of healthy libido.

But if you are often waking without an erection, this may indicate that the libido is too low, or that there may be an organic level of dysfunction – there may be some aspect of your 'plumbing' that is not working. If this is the case, and it is happening with regularity, I recommend you see your GP who may refer you to an andrologist or urologist.

Please be assured that ED is rife throughout our culture and GPs see many patients with this issue and indeed many doctors have a specialist interest in this subject. The NHS website and helpline provides information, and you may feel fully reassured that your doctor will maintain your confidentiality. Our libido is a very essential part of our health, and we should always pay attention to low libido as an indication that the stresses in our lives are imposing on our physiology.

When a man fails to get an erection, or struggles to maintain one, it can be just as inhibiting for the woman. Whereas he may be struggling with performance anxiety, she may also be feeling that she is not able to turn him on enough. So the performance issues of ED can make both of you feel insufficient and inhibited.

This is *not* a good recipe for the uninhibited lost-in-the-sensation lovemaking that is the very best place to be (whether you are trying to conceive or not). Unbidden sexual turn-on is one of the great delights of being, and should ideally arise without effort.

Then there is the case, when couples have been together for a long time, when habitual sex has become the norm, and spontaneity is not at the top of the agenda. A couple may have decentralised their sexual connection in favour of all the other rich aspects of their partnership. When the desire to become pregnant becomes the primary impetus for lovemaking, this may lead to an emotional political tangle.

So I would like you to reconsider how you can spice up your lovemaking with the things that really turn *your* cranks. This does require willingness and bravery to table your thoughts and feelings with each other, exploring what you would both like to try, seeking to sparkle your loving with what turns you on.

Being in the place of trying to express that you are not feeling the spontaneous desire of attraction is a very vulnerable place to be indeed. Yet, when you turn your hearts and minds to the reasons why you love each other, and approach these vulnerabilities from the space of the trust you have for each other, this will help to give you the foundation from which to re-kindle your desires.

If the issues between you as a couple have escalated to the point whereby you find it difficult or impossible to talk about sex, then I would urge you to think about finding a counsellor or sex therapist with whom you can unpack these vulnerable emotions in a safe and structured way. Sometimes it is easier to say the un-sayable in the presence of a qualified neutral third party who can listen without judgement and help you to find a way to communicate your fears and concerns with each other.

If you are seeking this kind of support, please be sure to look for a practitioner who has experience working with this particular kind of issue. Fertility Angst is a unique emotion and it is helpful to work with someone who has a strong understanding of the pressures and issues you are facing in this context of trying to conceive.

Sometimes this emotional tangle is the impediment that lies at the heart of not conceiving. We need to feel that we will be bringing a child into a relationship of trust and mutual support, knowing that the unconditional love you have for each other will be the linchpin of strength that will give you the ballast to parent your child together.

These can be very difficult things to offload. If the knots in your relationship are obstructing your sexual intimacy then I urge you to seek support to unwind them to find your way back into a loving exchange.

Performance anxiety

When I Google 'performance anxiety', the key advice is to 'reduce your stress'. This makes me cross. Most sites do not advise how to reduce that stress, or how to cope with the feelings of inadequacy that hit both partners when the erection is not 'woody' enough.

It is a good first port of call to sit down together to chat about what, within the context of your daily lives, is making you feel stressed. Can you find constructive ways in which you might change some of the habits and patterns in your life that generate or perpetuate your daily stresses? This might be as simple as really looking carefully at your diet. Remember the interrelationship of the digestive and sexual/reproductive hormones and the importance of a balanced blood sugar level to maintain good parasympathetic status – vital for a healthy libido.

Can you change your daily routine to simplify your travel/work pressures? Is there anything you can negotiate with your boss to ease the level of pressure you feel at work? If the work scenario isn't flexible, can you look at how you might shift the ways you are managing your leisure time? Can you create a leisure space that prioritises lovemaking and creates time for you to focus your energies towards each other?

The key is to work together to open up a space in your lives that is all about you as a couple and to make time for your lovemaking. This is tremendously important. Time and time again, I hear couples protest, 'no no, we are just too busy, too swamped with this commitment or that commitment' – *but* weirdly, if you found yourselves to be pregnant, suddenly those same impediments would be eminently changeable – and boy, does that baby take up a load of space!

So in this quest to alter the dynamics of your lives to reduce the stresses and strains of daily living when coupled within the journey to conceive, may I suggest you allow yourselves to relinquish the things that eat up your energies in a negative way.

Allow yourselves to make the space that an infant will require, and into that space throw your energies towards all the lovemaking, turn-each-other-on, shag-each-other-for-the-fun-of-it kind of sexual energy. Good loving will go a very long way to helping reduce your stress, especially when you are able to allow your lovemaking to have as much time as it needs.

Very often performance anxiety is related to an expectation of our lover's expectations of us, so we spend all our energies invested in the sympathetic response of believing that we are not good enough. The erection suffers, and she feels inadequate about not turning him on and he feels inadequate about not having the wood force that should be his innate sexual energy.

Whew.

Hand swipes brow as we all take a calming breath to recover from the hectic difficulty that all these emotional tangles engender. Tying in knots is never a good plan. Which brings us back to my frustration with the lack of good advice on the Internet for couples who are struggling with erectile dysfunction. This is a subject that has no easy arena for airing or treatment, and it is an arena that affects many couples.

Please don't avoid talking with each other about this. It is a *very* vulnerable place, and it does require a certain kind of courage. Your willingness to forgive each other for being human is the greatest kindness you can offer.

There is a strong component of inhibition and sense of insufficiency that will always accompany an erectile dysfunction, and there is only one way forward in the minefield: grab your magical landmine detector kit, take each other by the hand, put one foot forward and start finding your way, together, step by trepeditious step, back towards loving engagement.

Take the pressure off the penetrative sex, take the pressure off any need for there to be an erection. Just kiss and embrace. Just be together and try to open up all the things which may be causing the emotional tangles.

If it just seems too insurmountable to find your way into this tender conversation on your own, please look for a local practitioner who may be able to provide you both with the safety and structure of a therapeutic space to unwind your feelings. There are now many well-trained sexual therapists who have the sensitivity and experience to walk you safely through this minefield.

Be sure to find someone who has experience of working with couples who are having sexual issues coupled with experience of working with TTC issues.

Yang wilt

This is the Chinese medicine terminology for low libido, and it does do what it says on the box. Yang is the outward-bursting energy that is opposite of yin, the gathering inward deep energy. Most people these days have some sense of the idea of yin and yang. I have no desire to sound like a hippy-chick (though I will admit to Canadian west coast hippy roots) but the phrase *yang wilt* for me encapsulates what often happens in our culture.

Erectile dysfunction (ED) is a growing issue and affects men of many ages, tending to be more significant for men in their forties, fifties and sixties. Though saying that, the regular/excessive use of alcohol and the effects of recreational drugs, particularly cocaine, does take a significant toll, especially in combination with poor dietary habits, overwork and not enough rest. Many younger men in their twenties and thirties are struggling with episodic erectile dysfunction relating to drugs, alcohol, and to being over-stressed.

Do I need to mention again the effect of the stress hormones blocking the sexual hormones? When we are in an adrenalin cascade this will block our capacity to feel and respond to sexual excitement. Reducing stress is one of the fundamental approaches to building libido.

Yang wilt is slightly different from the ideas we have just discussed, whereby the erectile dysfunction may be related to a plumbing problem, or when the monkey brain gets in the way and performance anxiety is the core issue.

In yang wilt we are more specifically addressing why a man's yang energy, his thrusting power, may be compromised. It's not rocket science, and it's not news to all you TTC couples. The toll that modern life takes depletes our yang energy. Whether we are male or female, our libido is an expression of our yang energy. If a woman is struggling to feel a vibrant sexual desire, this too might be understood in this context of yang wilt, although women are much more complicated than men due to the cyclical fluctuation of hormone rhythms.

We have established the toll that modern life can take and we can see that diet, working hours, commute, sitting all day, the pressure of timing of our shagging, not conserving our reserves of energy, a lack of truly restful leisure, overly challenging exercise, toxins and electromagnetic over-exposure (for instance, to laptops, smart phones, tablets) can all significantly contribute to depleting our yang energies.

Usually all these things add up, a little here and a little there, culminating in an overall depletion of yang. It's that feeling of being tired all the time, and in our coffee culture we usually try to boost our yang throughout the day by using the uplift (yang) rush we get from caffeine and sugar.

Our libido is reliant upon how much reserve energy we hold, and modern life does indeed beat the crap out of our reserves. It is important in our efforts to improve our fertility that we pay primary attention to conserving our energy so that we can channel that surplus into the dynamic that is our sexual energy.

This is where the Chinese medicine diagnosis can really help. I would like to encourage all men and women who are feeling a lack of libido to consider the value of a course of Chinese medicine treatment. The diagnostic process of Chinese medicine can help to improve your reserve energies. Chinese medicine is much more than just acupuncture and herbs, and includes diet and lifestyle advice according to your Chinese constitutional diagnosis. We can help you to identify the taxations in your life that are depleting you, and can recommend the remedies that will help to replenish your reserves.

Acupuncture is all about energy: building deficiencies, clearing blockages, and resolving disharmonies. Chinese herbs can be a hugely beneficial way to bring in the medicinal components that help to improve your energy, not to mention how much they can improve sperm parameters and streamline menstrual function. This book is not intended as a guide to Traditional Chinese Medicine, but in the case of low libido I sincerely believe that TCM is one of the best therapies to improve your sexual dynamic.

Dynamic is the key word here. The more great sex that we have, the more we want; the more we think about it, the more we are stimulated.

We are ever the sum total of the marriage between our physical selves and our mind/heart. If low libido is an issue, look at all the ways in which your daily life may be putting strain and drain upon you. Examine where the downfall may be, always in the context of knowing that it is in the fine balance between the physical and the emotional that we function sexually.

Signs and symptoms that tell us our libido is low:

- Fatigue
- Weakness of the backs and knees
- Decreased morning erections
- Decreased firmness of erections
- Decreased orgasmic intensity

- No sexual thoughts during the day
- No unbidden desire to touch our lover.

'Grab and go' dietary habits that will lead to decreased libido:

- An erratic eating schedule
- Scant or no breakfast (a coffee and a Danish does not a breakfast maketh)
- Sandwiches for lunch in front of the computer
- Eating too much, too rich, too late in the evening.

I cannot emphasise enough how significantly our dietary habits will influence the hormonal triggers that govern our libidinous hormones. If we have an imbalance in our blood sugar levels this *will* affect our libido. We are what we eat, and what we eat hugely influences our sexual function. (More on this to come ...)

In trying to conceive the most important thing you can do is focus on your sexuality and do all that you can to build and develop your sexual energy.

Libido *is* the power of conception.

Women's libido

We have discussed at length the menstrual cycle and the ways in which daily life impacts on our hormonal fluctuations. Women's cycles are hugely influenced by the rhythms of nature, in particular the lunar cycle, the daily circadian rhythms (the sleep-wake cycle), and also our bio-rhythms, which are a combination of our mental, physical and emotional activity. We may also be influenced by seasonal fluctuations and the changing cosmos – how and where the stars and planets are at any given time within the calendar.

Whether or not you may ascribe to any of these ideas, the reality of our humanness is that we are mammals within the animal kingdom, and as such we are subject to the laws of nature. And women are very much subject to the rhythms of nature, as our menstruation is a cycle that is hugely influenced by the gravitational ebb and flow of the lunar cycle.

Learning about our specific menstrual cycle is an important part of understanding ourselves as women, never more important than when we are trying to conceive. As women come on their period, this is the time for hand jobs and blow jobs, a non-sexual time. Meaning, that this is not the optimum time for a woman to be bringing her body into a state of sexual excitement, as it's busy sorting out the menstruation – hence, focus on his pleasure.

As the period finishes and the endometrium is building, the oestrogen is rising, the follicle is growing. We turn a tide to flow towards the peak that is ovulation, and shift back towards our sexuality. The busyness of the period is over, and now our body has that surplus of energy to turn towards lovemaking. This week before ovulation is a great time for vigorous adventurous experimental no-holds-barred shagging!

Just before the ovulation, as we come on to the stretchy mucus, as the LH surge is building and releasing, we are at our most oestrogenic. This should be a horny time. In the same way that NPT, the morning glory, is a sign of healthy male libido, a vibrant sexual wanting just before ovulation is a good sign of female libido. We are slippery with our spinn mucus, we are glowing on the vibrancy that is a full dose of oestrogen, our pheromones are blasting, we should very much *desire* sexual contact at this time.

If you are coming towards your ovulation with get-outta-my-face PMS-like symptoms, this is, unfortunately, not very healthy. Feeling too emotional, tearful, frustrated, short-tempered or downright angry around the ovulation is your body's way of suggesting that your sexual energy is compromised.

If you are feeling like this, please do not beat yourself up. This is a kind of equivalent yang wilt, essentially a female ED. It simply means the energetic powerhouse that nourishes your libido is depleted. Very often this lack of energy has to do with your input-output ratios, and by increasing good foods and qualitative rest you can help replenish the deficiencies that are undermining your sexuality.

Girls, the follicular phase is a time for you to be very focused on the things that bring you pleasure – and I ain't talkin' about shopping! This is a time to be thinking about *sex*, to be considering what makes you turn on, to be focused on seducing your lover and teaching him what you would like to do sexually that really makes you hot.

If the disharmonies in your menstrual cycle are giving you PMS-like symptoms that are inhibiting your sexual triggers, then this should be understood to be pathological. That is not a scary word, it simply means 'not in correct function'. So if you are feeling non-sexual leading into ovulation, this is your body telling you that you are experiencing stresses and strains.

I urge you to examine your daily life and find the ways to open the doorway into your sexuality. I cannot recommend Chinese medicine diagnosis highly enough as a powerful tool to helping you to do this.

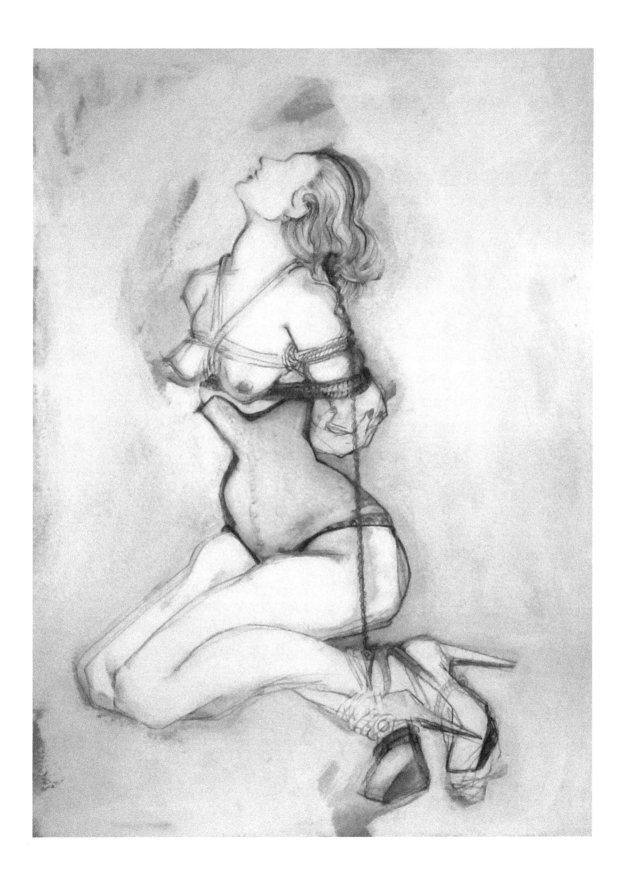

all that we can be

i love that you love this
that binding is your thing
being tied is, always has been
my favourite fantasy
yet
i have never had a lover who has taken me there
in the way that i wish for

for the first time i truly understand how a hard-on must feel for a man
because the way this affects me
imagining you doing these things to me
the clenchsqueezepull feeling that it brings
so bursting with ache
so desperate for touch
must be the sensation of a full and straining cock

and when i feel this
and imagine you feeling it too
then the surge blasts harder and i just WANT even more

i so hope it pleases you
to know what you are doing this to me
i hope that it makes you feel even more avaricious
that it pushes you to greater lengths
of letting yourself go

to the place where your desires will lead you
unbidden
unleashed
unruly
unrestrained
undulations
of horniness

which is why you must tie me down
in order to anchor
this wave of unfettered exploration

a point of attachment from which to let go

i long for your touch
for your kiss
for your tenderness
and
for your fierceness

come and let yourself be
with me
to be
all that we can be

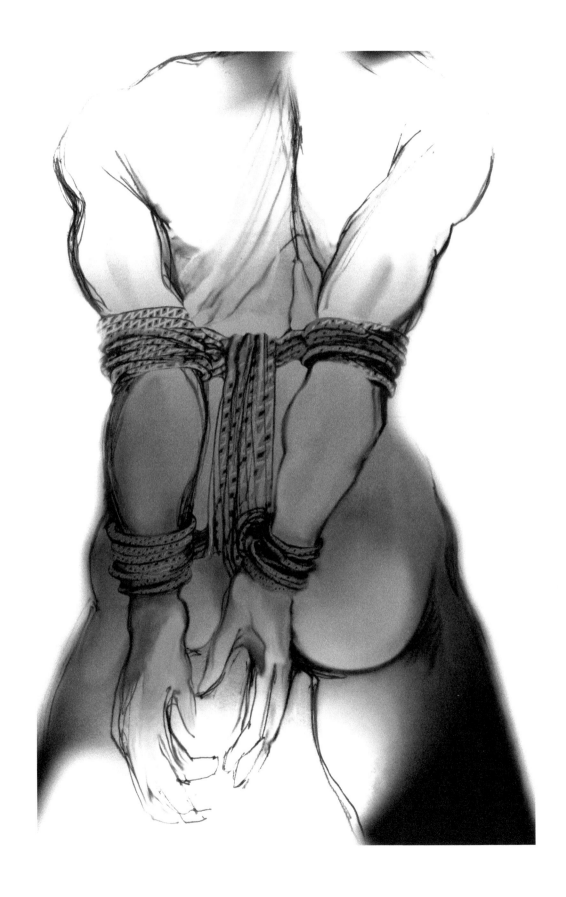

Chapter Ten

Guilt and blame – his and hers

This bit is one of the simplest, and one of the most difficult challenges.

Simple?! Ohh come on Jani! How can this fundamentally thorny issue be deemed as simple?

Well, here's me with that Chinese Medicine Hat on again. For in Chinese medicine we understand how easily sperm parameters can be improved. How easily menstrual function can be improved. How wonderful Assisted Conception can be when it has the capacity to take us past an insurmountable physiologic challenge.

Whether the issue is due to male or female factor reason, or, if you are lost in that swamp of the non-diagnosis that is 'unexplained infertility', we do know that good diet and improvements to lifestyle can hugely improve fertile parameters. Add in some regular acupuncture and herbal or nutritional supplementation, and the likelihood is that we will see even more improvement. Especially if we reduce that switchy chronic stress response mechanism I've mentioned (once or twice ...).

Where it gets difficult is in the unspoken hindrances that can develop between a couple at the level of guilt and blame.

Female factor: Month after month there is no conception. No matter how hard she tries, no matter how diligently perfect her lifestyle changes are, no matter how much she strives to hope, period after period comes, or month after month there is no ovulation, and time and time again she feels undermined as a woman, incapable of stepping into the destiny that she believes is her purpose in life.

Male factor: His sense of inadequacy may lead towards the erectile dysfunction of monkey brain getting in the way, as he feels unable to satisfy his lover on multiple levels. She feels unfulfilled and confused, she loses confidence that he finds her attractive, everyone is unhappy.

Each may be blaming the other for not being able to make a baby, and then feeling guilty as hell for such a damningly negative thought about the one they love.

A recipe for an emotional tangle if ever there was one.

There is only one way forward through this minefield: you simply (this is the most *difficult* bit) must be able to *talk* with each other. Honest expression of your true heart feelings will help you through this particular difficulty. I want to assure you that these thoughts and feelings of guilt and blame are normal.

Please cut yourselves some slack. Instead of putting all your energy into feeling these negative thoughts, try to re-examine *all* the aspects of your daily life and support each other in generating the changes that will help to improve your sperm and eggs. Remember, oxytocin is the bonding hormone. The very first instance you clapped eyes on each other it was the dopamine/oxytocin cascades that ruled your coming together.

Bring your energy back into that attraction and you will significantly diminish these negative feelings. Allowing that you have these negative feelings is a very important part of working through this. Many people avoid admitting that guilt and blame is at the heart of what they are feeling, so do please let your honest emotions flow, for in being honest you will be able to resonate in your truth. And when you stand in your truth, then you are three-quarters of the way to a resolution.

The emotions around not conceiving are deeply scary. The best advice I can offer you is to not turn away from each other when these horrible emotions get in the way. By owning the way you are feeling you stand every chance of stepping past the barriers that guilt and blame engender. By willingly acknowledging that this is standing in your heart, you stand every chance of melting it away through the power of love.

Egads, I hate to sound like some kind of evangelical preacher! But truly, I am speaking to you from the heart – this is one of the most miraculous aspects of being human. Love does conquer all. When the emotions of not conceiving begin to stand in the way of you and your lover, then the only way back is through the willingness to be true to each other. This is the pillar of a good relationship.

Simply, the most difficult challenge.

If these issues feel too big to tackle, too overwhelming, too intense, too vulnerable, too scary – look for a good person with whom you can safely unpack these emotional knots. There are so many great therapists out there, so find someone who has experience working with TTC couples.

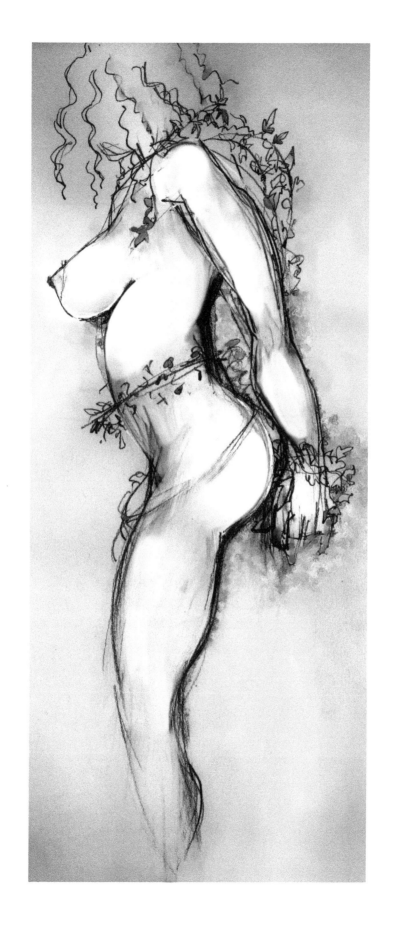

apology

my words hurt you
cut your confidence like a knife

you say that no words can heal this
that you will only believe my regret
through conviction of genuine touch

you are far away now
but if i was with you …

i would take your cheeks softly into my hands
relishing the rasp of your stubble on my skin
as i turn your head to look me square on
sinking my gaze
as deeply as a well of pure spring water of inky black unfathomable depths
and as i draw you into my gaze
the lightness of clear heart shining a smile of simple joy directly into you
my hands will tendril up to twist the soft soft loveliness of your beautiful hair
my questing fingers drawing your head to mine
feather light
to dance my breath upon your welcome
to open the heart space between us
as
with the softest of apologies
i kiss you

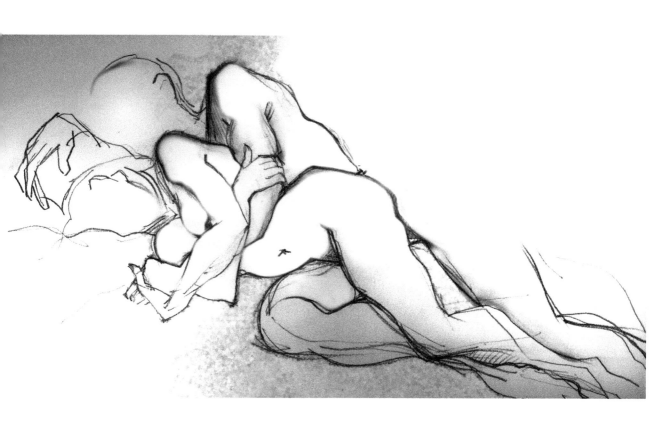

Chapter Eleven

Seasonal rhythms

One aspect of modern life that drains our reserves is that we no longer live such seasonal lives. We have a much more 24/7 approach these days, anything goes, any time.

Did you know that the highest success rates in IVF always happen in April–May? (Oct–Nov in the Southern Hemisphere). That's nature for you! The bursting, sap-rising energies of spring are all about germination, budding, opening, blossoming. It makes sense that IVF results also rise at this time of year, as the energies of birth are the predominant force within nature's rhythms in the spring.

Seasonal energies do influence us, and sadly we are creating a predominantly urban lifestyle that on some levels allows us to ignore these natural rhythms. We are living in a sort of bubble, whereby we can live by the same rhythms all day, all through the year. Whether it be winter, spring, summer or autumn, our routines are determined by our work schedules rather than the prevailing climate and the movement of the sun – whereas ideally we should have shorter working days in the winter, longer days in the summer.

Nowadays, we tend to have as social a time in the winter as we would in the summer. Although it is actually only one day, Christmas has turned December (and November, and now even *October)* into the most hectic period of the year, as we run around like crazy to fit in all the retail-orientated festivities and social commitments. Rather than have a slower time with longer sleeps in the winter, we often socialise as we would during the height of summer.

This also applies to the gym-fit approach to exercise. Rather than allowing the weather to dictate the type of exercise we choose, we roll on with the same output regardless of the time of year. When we lose the conserving power that a slow approach gives us during the winter months, we come into the spring with less reserves, for we haven't used the winter's time to replenish our energies.

In addition, we control our environments in such a way that it is harder for our bodies to be in tune with the seasonal fluctuations. We move from our centrally heated homes to our centrally heated offices, which are cooled with air conditioning in the summer, maintaining a consistent temperate zone no matter what the weather, no matter what the season.

Seasonal fluctuations are an important part of the rhythms of nature and help to govern our hormonal fluctuations. Conserving our energies through the winter brings us the oomph and burst of rising spring energies, followed by the warmth of expansiveness that is the summer, back into the gentle contraction of autumn.

I'm not asking you to go back to living on the land, in tune with every nuance of the natural world. But I am asking if you need to go hammer and tongs at an unvarying pace all the year long, give some thought as to how you might bring a better seasonal awareness into your daily life.

One of the important things you can do in your efforts to bring your body, mind and heart into its most fertile capacity is to spend as much time as you can out of doors. Nature is a great leveller. She will always show us who is fundamentally in control, and her power is awe-inspiring. Connecting with nature will help you to connect with the power of fecundity.

If you are lucky enough to have a lovely park nearby, try a regular walk during your lunch break. Not only will you benefit your circulatory systems, you will notice seasonal fluctuations. Like listening to music, nature bathes our senses and brings us into the calm of parasympathetic, aiding our hormone flows to do what they should be doing.

Just like the birds and bees.

Circadian rhythms

Many people habitually stay up too late, instead of bringing themselves down into the restful replenishment of quality sleep. (Here we go again ... I'm banging that drum.) The power for conception is predicated on our reserves, ergo, the more we replenish our energy, while conserving our output, the better our reserves will be. You will really begin to make headway when you find that your replenishments (the right kind of diet, exercise, and rest for you) begin to outweigh your taxations – then you will begin to gain some ground.

And while I'm banging this drum, can we please recognise that all of this is in the context of *normal daily life*. I do not advocate that you become some kind of Zen-Hero! I'm suggesting that with mindfulness, being aware of what drains you and what nourishes you, you can begin to hugely increase your fertile capacities. Cherry-pick the replenishments that work for you, ditch the things which tax your energy, always in the context that there is no need to do it all at once.

Your circadian rhythms are your sleep/wake cycle, and are governed by the hormones serotonin and melatonin.

There is ever-growing concerns about the issue of blue light, as all of our device screens, TVs, computers, tablets, Kindles and mobile phones emit it, as do energy-saving light bulbs. It is this blue light that boosts our attention, enhances alertness and increases reaction time during the day, but blue light also inhibits the production of melatonin, the hormone that triggers us to sleep. There is growing evidence that a link exists between evening screen use and insomnia.

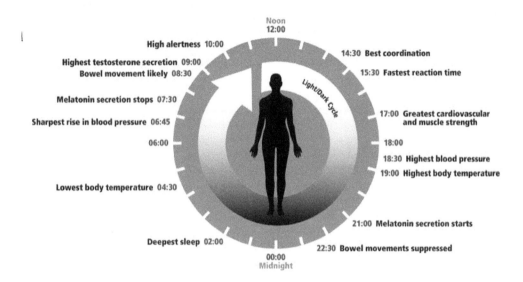

Noon
12:00

High alertness 10:00

Highest testosterone secretion 09:00
Bowel movement likely 08:30

Melatonin secretion stops 07:30

Sharpest rise in blood pressure 06:45

06:00

Lowest body temperature 04:30

Deepest sleep 02:00

00:00
Midnight

14:30 Best coordination

15:30 Fastest reaction time

17:00 Greatest cardiovascular
and muscle strength

18:00

18:30 Highest blood pressure
19:00 Highest body temperature

21:00 Melatonin secretion starts

22:30 Bowel movements suppressed

Light/Dark Cycle

From Environmental Health Perspectives 2010 Jan; Vol 118; 1.

Serotonin and melatonin regulate the sleep/wake cycle, and they regulate mood and appetite and sleep. If our body clock is disrupted by thinking that the night is the day, this swings our whole circadian rhythm out of balance.

The disruption of the serotonin and melatonin balance will have a knock-on effect throughout our digestive feedback loops; and as 90 per cent of serotonin is produced in the gut, this will also affect the balance of our sexual and reproductive hormones.

The beauty of our autonomic nervous system is the exquisite interplay of the feedback loops that consistently strive to ensure that we are always in the optimum state of rest and digest – the state that best enhances our fertility. I'm always impressed by just how much pressure our bodies can take and still retain that balance.

It is a measure of how stressful our modern living is that 30 per cent of couples are diagnosed with unexplained infertility. Personally I would much rather change that to 'sub-fertility due to alterations in the finely tuned homeostatic balance of the digestive and reproductive hormone balances'. Somehow doubt that phrase will catch on, but for you, dear reader, I request that you grasp on to this understanding that each and every little thing you can do to ease the stresses your system is under *will* help to enhance your fertile capacities.

So why is it important to be in bed before 11 p.m.?

The power of TCM

This part is also to do with Chinese medicine (I know this *isn't* a Traditional Chinese Medicine book, but there are so many things I really want to share). I just can't help myself – I've seen so many hundreds of couples benefit from the most *simple changes*.

One of the very most important aspects of TCM diagnosis and treatment is the diet and lifestyle advice and guidance specific to your constitution. A constitutional diagnosis helps you to find the right foods, the right cooking methods, the right exercise and the right kind of rest *for you*. A TCM diagnosis will also help you to recognise what is taxing your energies and the appropriate ways to replenish those energies.

Correct diet, correct exercise and correct rest are *primary* replenishments. Acupuncture and herbs are the secondary replenishments that will enhance these dietary and lifestyle changes.

We humans are an amazing orchestration of immense complexity. Correct diet, exercise and rest are vital to our well-being, and they are vital to healthy conception. Our libido relies on our vitality. Building good vitality aids a healthy conception, promotes a glowing pregnancy, facilitates a gentle delivery and enhances a strong recovery.

The primary power to replenish and build your fertility is in your own capable hands.

We have a saying in TCM that when you are horizontal 'the blood returns to the organs'. When we are lying down all the blood and fluids have a chance to move from the peripheries, the arms and legs, to the centre, back into the organs of the abdominal and chest cavities. Your organs are like the ministry offices within the state-like structure that is your body, ie. they are the place where the decisions are made.

In TCM the word 'blood' includes all the plasma, the lymph and the interstitial fluids that move through all the systems of your body, not just the arterial and venous blood circulation. Interstitial means the spaces between all the membranes, muscles, and sinews – which is quite *a lot* of space – did you know that the human body is 70.8 per cent fluid? It is through all these fluids that the molecular hormonal messages that move via neurotransmission are shunted around your systems, allowing your parasympathetic to keep you breathing and digesting and reproducing.

In TCM we refer to 12 channel (or meridian) systems to describe the planes of the human body, so when TCM says 'Liver' or 'Kidney' or 'Spleen', we mean the *channel system* that has that name. We relate the circadian rhythms to the body's channel systems. Each of the channels have a 2-hour slot where they are the dominant system. For example between 11 p.m. to 3 a.m. the dominant channel systems are the paired Gall Bladder and Liver.

The liver organ is important for our hormonal balance because it plays a *huge* role in the detoxification of the body, and in TCM we understand that this detox process primarily happens during the 11 p.m. to 3 a.m. time slot – *but* it only happens if we are horizontal. If we are up and buzzing about, our blood is in the peripheries. If we are at the computer, our blood is in the peripheries. If we are sitting up in bed, reading or watching TV, the blood is in the peripheries.

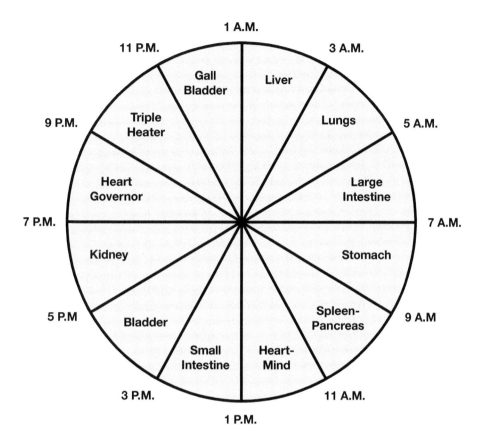

If we are horizontal, all those fluids, the plasma, the lymph, the interstitials, the red blood cells, the white blood cells, return to centre, to be moved through the liver to be cleaned and divided up into either the waste systems and to be re-circulated into the body. When this function is happening appropriately we feel revitalised, we gain better quality sleep, and we wake with a vibrancy in our systems.

This clean-up process is vital to the smooth movement of the hormonal messaging in our systems. It's simple, really: efficient daily detoxification during those 11 p.m. to 3 a.m. hours of appropriate (horizontal) liver function makes us healthier. If you would like to improve the quality of your rest, and to aid your systems into more optimum function, then ensure you are tucked up in bed by around 10.30 p.m.

In respect of blue light, the advice from Harvard Medical School is to turn your screens off 90 minutes before you go to bed. So the ideal recipe is switch off the electrics by 9 p.m. and be in bed for 10.30 p.m. This may seem like a difficult ask, for most of us do tool around with a screen in the evening, and most of us do stay up quite late. As ever, let's look at this in bite-sized chunks.

I challenge you to try this for just one week, and in doing so evaluate how it affects your quality of energy and your quality of sleep. And hey! Just think about how much lovemaking time you create by not wasting away hours on Facebook ...

Simple things can make the most significant differences.

This book is all about the things you can do in your own home, at your own hearth, in the privacy of your own love life, and it's very much in the context of ring fencing your rest time and generating a powerful work/life balance. My ambition is to help point you towards the choices that work for you, to help you find the ways to take control of the way you are managing your lives, and it is all about helping you find ways that you can build your reserves and minimise your taxations.

Electro disruption

In the context of building up good-quality replenishing sleep, I ask you to consider removing all the electronic devices from your bedroom. Electronic energy imposes a counterproductive influence on our bodies. Like the planet, our bodies have a north/south polarity, which means that we are orientated to a vertical exchange of energies throughout the body. Electromagnetic energy has a horizontal wave.

When we are in front of the TV, at the computer, on the laptop or tablet or phone, we are imposing that horizontal pull against our vertical polarity. This is another of the very key reasons why we are all so tired all the time, as our bodies need to work harder to maintain normal function.

My plea is to recognise that we are under this electronic influence virtually all the time now, and now we suffer the influence of WiFi virtually everywhere we go.

Consider making your bedroom into a sanctuary, where none of this influence will be emitting rays while you sleep. In my humble opinion, bedrooms should be for *lovemaking* and for *sleeping*, and nothing else. It may be of huge benefit to reconfigure your space so that it is all about, and only about, sex and sleep.

Another good habit is to switch the sockets off at the wall, so that there is no live current in your space.

Watching television/films just before bed activates the brain, as does any engagement with an electronic device. The effort our brains need to make in order to turn those thousands of pixels into images and words makes them very active indeed. A major component of sleep is the need for the brain to switch off, to allow those zillions of synapses to have a rest. Booting up your brain activity just before sleep is not helpful.

So, take the trappings of daily life out of your bedchamber and put the lovemaking emphasis into your bedrooms. Monitor for yourself to see if just removing the electronics doesn't improve the quality of your sleep. Add to that getting horizontal before 11 p.m., and you should see an increase in your vitality, and with that a most beneficial charge to your sexual energies.

Taking away the electro will charge up your lovemaking!

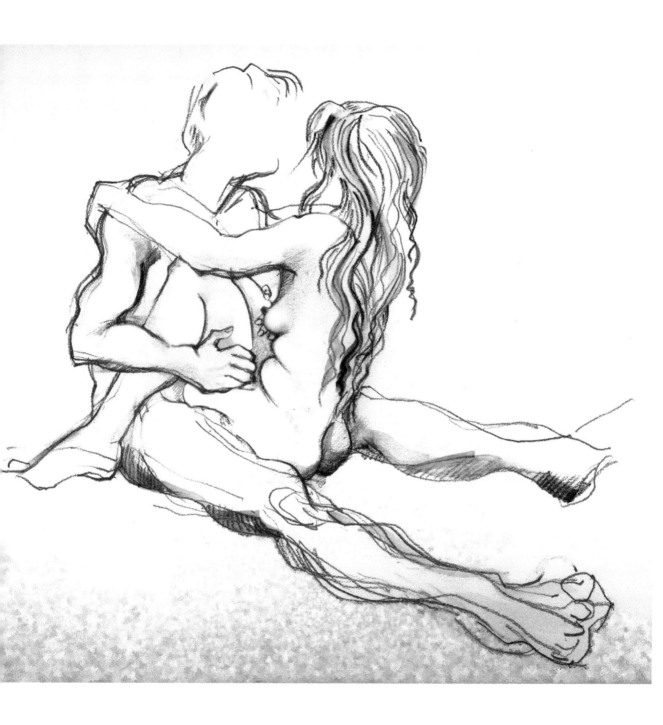

almost kiss

the way you almost kissed me
lips held but millimetres apart
no contact
and yet
sheer eroticism of shared breath
so fraught with potential of passion

i stepped away in a daze of wanting
dizzy with the desire to know more
to feel how you feel
to feel you feel me
peel me
unveil me

layer by layer
to discover each other

knowing well
that here is a lover
with whom one may trust

for in trust
boundaries dissolve
to limitless horizons
opening to a sea of ardour
oceans deep endless skies
with routes to map
lands to find

a place to be
to just be

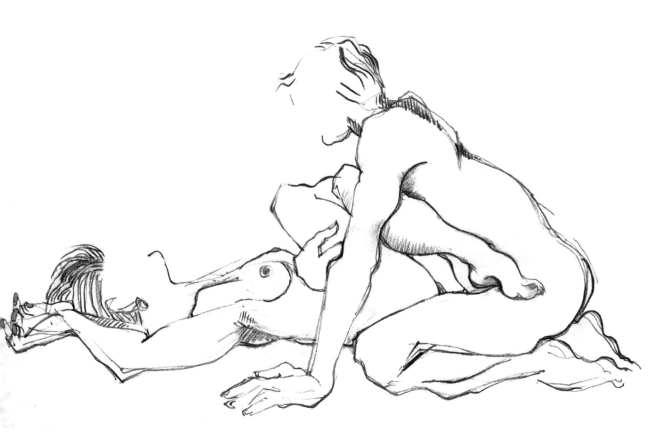

Chapter Twelve

Exercise

We live in a culture whereby 'fitness' is deemed to be of paramount importance. And it is. Our culture of sitting, of wrong foods, of over consumption, is leading to all kinds of health problems. But it is important to ask ourselves what it really means to be fit. For many people this is defined by body image, not by actual wellness.

Being fit is not just about having a toned body. Genuine fitness comes from having systems that are working well; an efficient metabolism, good circulation, lots of blood and fluids moving through the muscle and sinews, efficient digestion and reproductive fluency, healthy libido and natural vitality.

Many people find it difficult to exercise in the context of the work/commute grind, and feel that if they are not regularly going to the gym/swim/run/yoga/whatever, somehow they are not exercising; and if they do not have the airbrushed beautiful body that is so endemic in our media culture then they are not fit enough.

This book is a mantra for helping you to find the ways to bring your body into the peak of its own specific capacities. For many people, the exercise regime they choose may be depleting rather than enlivening them. It can be tricky to unwind this notion.

Many of us have quite sedentary lives and feel much better after we do a workout, as the buzz of endorphins and increased circulation create a sense of well-being that helps us to feel better. But sometimes this feeling is a mask, and we are mistaking the initial endorphin high for a feeling of genuine *wellness*.

Many of us approach exercise from a place of being under-powered, where our reserves are already lowered. Sometimes a strict exercise regime can actually deplete us further.

Am I being clear? Exercise is good and it is important for our wellness. It's just that for many of us, the kind of exercise we choose is not necessarily the kind of exercise that is actually nourishing *our* body.

Rest is an important and *valuable* part of our wellness. When it comes to exercise the important thing to evaluate is not so much how you feel immediately after your workout, but to carefully consider how it makes you feel the next day.

Does the exercise bring you better energy? Do you sleep better? Do you wake feeling refreshed? Does it enliven you? Does it increase your libido? Or, does your exercise regime actually drain you? This is a vital question to ask. The gym-fit approach may sometimes tax you rather than nourish you.

There are many ways to exercise. I cannot emphasise enough the value of walking, of swimming and of cycling (not necessarily spinning!). The reason I like to suggest these forms of exercise is that they can get you outside (try walking to the pool) into the fresh air, into the seasons, and you are able to easily *modulate* how you are exercising.

It is important to be able to choose the pace you are working at. This is why spinning can be so taxing: it may pressurise you to maintain a pace that will demand more than your reserves can offer.

Walking is absolutely marvellous, and running (if that's your thing – personally, don't get it), is a great way to get out and moving, but at the same time allows you to modulate the pace according to how your energy is in the moment. Some days you may be feeling bright energy and feel inclined to move at a ferocious pace that gets your heart really pumping. Other days, you may benefit from just taking a stroll, moving your muscles, circulating your blood, but at a pace that acknowledges your body is really tired.

So give yourself permission to take your exercise at your own pace, respect your fluctuating energy levels and always listen carefully to the messages that your body is giving you.

The gym-style regime of exercise can sometimes be an added pressure on us to push our body beyond where it needs to be, plus the gym keeps us indoors. One of the huge benefits of exercising outdoors is that it really helps your body to attune to the seasons: a gentler pace in the winter, a vibrant acceleration in the spring, building to a height of movement in the summer, slowing again as the autumn brings you back into winter.

Going hammer and tongs all the way through the seasons, at the same pace throughout the year, is not a healthy way to live our lives.

Yoga and Pilates are a vitally important part of looking at what fitness really means. In both of these disciplines we find the only kinds of exercise that move the muscles fibres in both a longitudinal and latitudinal way. These exercise regimes help to improve circulation by helping the body to release the lactic acids that accumulate in the muscle fibres (an off-shoot of the sympathetic response, as the body can over-produce lactic acids to counteract excess adrenalin).

Being supple is much more important than being toned. Our suppleness is a vital part of our ability to have babies, and this is just as important for men as women. Our sexuality requires a good degree of suppleness. And I promise you, the workout of lovemaking is by far the best way to get your body circulating, helping to zing the blood and fluids throughout your body, and in particular throughout your pelvic cavity, helping to create the sort of healthy environment that is welcoming to conception.

So please be mindful to choose workouts that really benefit you and do not over-tax your systems, and ensure that you are replenishing and building your energy rather than draining it.

Rest and leisure

We have reached a funny (odd, not ha ha) time in our society whereby we are moving at a pace that has hitherto been unknown to man. Never mind cars, trains and aeroplanes, think about the hyper-warp speed of the average infomercial, and the way technology moves information through the ether, dropping instantaneous communication into our very palms.

We are connected at all times, across the planet, through time zones, and over seas that previously took months to cross. I often wonder what it would be like to transport someone from nineteenth-century London and teleport them into Oxford Circus, central London on a Saturday afternoon. I suspect they would spend the whole time in a state of fear in the face of the sheer volume and speed of people. If they could experience the Internet and mobile phones I'm sure they would believe it was all supernatural.

Most of us do move through a relatively hectic world and hardly notice at all just how it assaults our senses. It is because we are so accustomed to this fast pace, it has become normal. We are inured to the tempo at which we live our daily lives.

I believe this is partly why we feel so tired most of the time. Whenever I am lecturing I like to ask the assembled audience if there is anyone present who *doesn't* feel tired most of the time, keeping in mind that my audience is usually made up of healthcare professionals. Once in a blue moon a lone hand might appear, and invariably they do not live in a city.

What I would like to ask now is that you give some thought to the definition of rest and what it means to you, and that you consider the real difference between rest and leisure. We might plan to visit friends or go on a picnic or to an event, and we schlep through the required travel, maybe rushing about preparing the meal we will share, or dashing to fit in the housekeeping so that we can then go off to the outing. Often our 'time off' creates its own kind of hectic.

Do you take enough time to just do nothing? Do you let yourself have leisurely lie-ins and wake naturally? Do you let yourself have a bit of a lounge about, no plans, just drifting through the day, a bit of this, a bit of that, able to move with whim?

Or, if you do have a list of tasks, do you set enough time to be able to do them slowly in that ambling sort of way? Or is the DIY, supermarket shop, errands list jammed to the hilt so that you spend from 9–5 meeting all your retail ambitions on Saturday, and then spend all of Sunday doing the leisure activities that you shopped for?

The reason I want to ask these questions is that most of us think of our leisure time as rest time. BUT, we need to ask ourselves if this time off from our work lives is actually *restful*.

I often find, when I ask people how they spend their leisure time, that it includes a scheduled, relatively hurried, day. Going on holiday can be even *more* hectic, creating a compressed schedule to get everything done in order to get away, arrive, unpack, unwind, hit the chill zone and then it's time to pack for the reverse journey of similar travel slog, only to come back to twice as much work, as it has all piled up while we are supposedly 'off'.

Am I chiming any bells? Not to mention that many of us no longer switch off entirely, as we are still in mobile, email, Skype contact no matter where we are, and often our time 'away' is interspersed with the connection back into our work life.

When we are trying to conceive, *REST* is one of the most vital replenishments we can stoke up on. So in the same way that we can begin to develop a mindfulness about our nutritional input, of being aware of the right kinds of exercise without overdoing it, and getting the most beneficial kind of sleep, we can also turn our attention to taking a restful approach to our leisure time.

Ring-fencing and pyjama days

One of the key things you can do to help create this kind of restful leisure time is to begin 'ring-fencing' your time off.

You might begin by consciously loading less into your weekend. Why not prioritise to just do only one thing? Or perhaps a sequence of activities that gently flow into each other, rather than commitments that force you to move in 3 different directions. Cultivate an ambling pace with no time pressures.

Another suggestion would be that you only plan events for every other weekend, and to consciously close the doors to other commitments: put up a fence around your time for you and your partner to be together in a space with no schedule.

One of the things that we do rarely is to rest *responsively*. Meaning that we rarely allow ourselves to respond when our body is giving us signals to please just lie down and do nothing. By allowing ourselves to have a fully ring-fenced weekend we create the space and place for that kind of responsive resting.

By ring fencing, we can create a space where there is no pressure to do anything at all. Not only does this give us a marvellous chance to replenish our energies, but it also gives us a golden opportunity to put some of that replenishment into our sexual lives. It helps to create a wonderful space to seduce our lover in the luxury of one's own sweet time. And oh my, there is nothing so lovely as leisurely lovemaking followed by a most blissful oxytocin-satiated afternoon nap!

Ring-fencing is about creating a dedicated time to be with each other, without any agenda at all, allowing yourselves the richness of time to renew and restore your energies. One of the lovely things in a ring-fenced weekend, aside from leisurely shagging, is to amble into a market to buy fresh, vibrant foods, and to focus on cooking up some delicious recipes that will see you through the week. Instead of a sandwich scoffed at lunchtime in front of the computer you could be eating happy food that will nourish your fertility. We are what we eat, so stoking up on sex-fuelled nutrition has to be a good thing!

A pyjama day is an intervention that I created in one of the busiest times of my own life, when I was writing an MA programme, lecturing, running a full-time clinic and mothering my 2 boys. I began to realise that I was burning out, as most of the teaching was at weekends, thus I was working 7 days a week, writing until midnight every night, bang awake at 6.45 a.m. to get the kids off to school. Trust me – I know a thing or two about the values of ring-fencing!

I was going at my life so hammer and tongs, like the berloody clappers, that I knew I was going to go bust. So I invented:

The laws of pyjama day

1. you have to stay in your pyjamas all day
2. if you are in your pyjamas you are not allowed to do any housework
3. *under no circumstances* can you switch on the computer – any email, Skype, Facebook or any other computer-related communication is forbidden – and the Internet is fully off limits
4. mobile phones are switched off and no business calls can be made

5. duvet on the couch, movies, novels, magazines and naps are the order of the day

6. if you do need to go to the shops for a pint of milk – or, in my case, to walk the dogs – you have to go in your pyjamas – that's the rule. (All the people in my village came to know the laws of pyjama day and would cheerily greet me without batting an eye as I dropped into the local shop in my flannels, or trumped through the woods with said flannels tucked in my wellies)

7. it is permissible to eat quality prepared foods, ideally something you can pull out of the freezer that is on your nutritious list, but serious cooking is not allowed

8. scrambled eggs, bowls of cereal, cheese on toast, one long day of snacking is entirely permissible, meals are unnecessary

9. lie-ins, naps and long hot baths are de rigueur.

Pyjama days are a way of taking a step beyond ring-fencing, for those times when we realise that we are truly feeling exhausted. I highly recommend this fabulous way of rekindling one's mojo. Oh yeah, rule 10) after a day of rest and a long hot bath, shagging is totally on the permissible list.

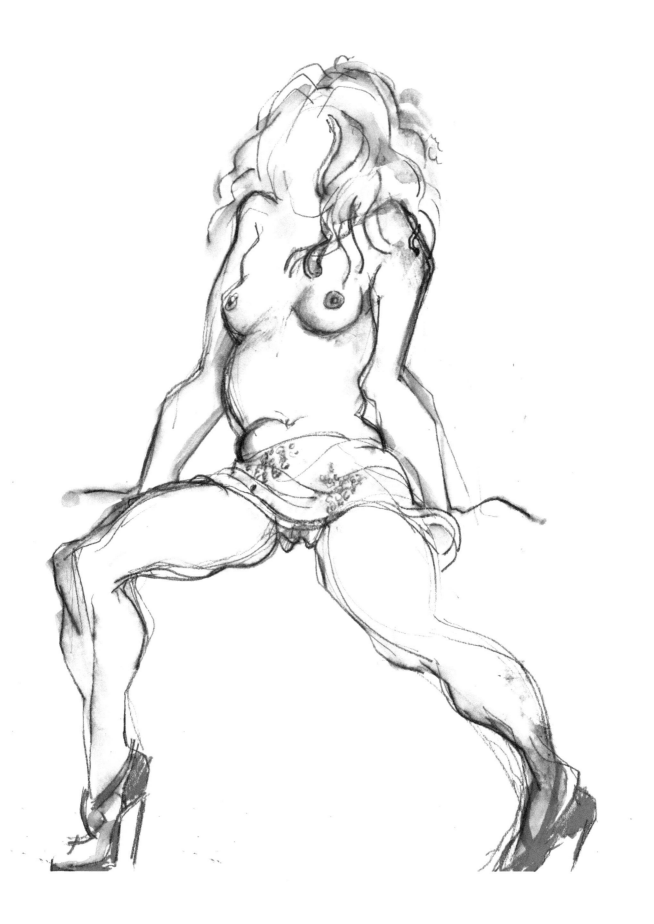

waterfall

on bended knee
you take my throbbing erect clit in your mouth
sucking me
hard sharp absolute
drowning me in the vortecy of your pulling draw
swallowing me whole
spiralling me down
velvet whirlpool

gently
swirling your tongue
soft sweet relief
then suddenly
flashing
between suck and swirl
hard and soft
clamping my hips in your arms
forcing my pelvis hard into your face
as i buck against the force of your mouth upon my button
my head thrashing
trying not to implode within the force of your force

with ardour
breath ragged
you jam your fingers into me
feeling how hot
how wet i am
as slowly you begin to fill me

finger by finger
widening me
pressing hard up into me
gypsy fingers sweet gypsy fingers
dancing your fingers within

you hook and pull
to feel the drench as i gush down onto you
waterfalling down your arm
all the pent of the previous moments
flooding my wanting onto you
hot hot waterfall of wanting

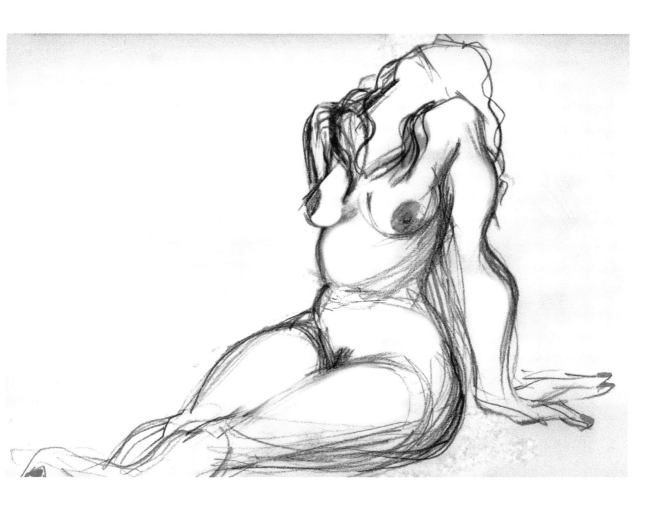

Chapter Thirteen

Everyone but me is pregnant

This is one of the worst things about trying to conceive, the noticing that *everyone* else seems to be falling pregnant, everyone has big bumps, is holding a newborn, is pushing that pushchair.

There is the dreaded family party, the wedding, the birthday, when Great Aunty Sally blurts out in front of everyone 'so when are you going to have a baby dearie, we're all waiting.' The girls in the office who one by one go off on maternity leave; the circle of close friends, who were also struggling, who, one by one, announce that they have conceived; the best friend who is worried about telling you her good news.

All the while you feel yourself in a quagmire of conflicting emotions. For though you are genuinely happy for your friend/sister/work colleague, you still can't help the surge of jealousy, envy, frustration, anger and fear.

These horrid emotions, please let me assure you, are *completely normal.*

One of the things about this journey of trying to conceive is to allow yourself the slack you will need to cope with all the negative emotions on this roller coaster ride. Please feel reassured that you can feel both happy for your friend and at the same time teeth-grittingly angry that it isn't happening for you. Why wouldn't the cold snake of fear not do a dance in your belly?

I want to reassure you that it is OK and very *normal* to feel these difficult emotions. What you don't want is for these feelings to become a stressful impediment to your well-being and your peace of mind.

Retaining some perspective is one of the most difficult aspects of the fertility journey. Month after month it still isn't happening, and we begin to castigate ourselves for feeling so jealous and angry and fearful, and we prefer to avoid the occasions when Great Aunty Sally will be present, and we no longer want to hang out with our friends because they all have bumps and we don't … *This* is when the impediment has set up camp and pulls you into that unhealthy switchy mechanism that can inhibit the free flow of oxytocin.

Find the courage to embrace the negative emotions that arise when you are faced with the 'everyone but me' factor. They aren't pretty, but they're yours. And by willingly accepting that these are normal responses, I hope that it will go a very long way to helping you to realise that, although you are in a complicated place, you will neutralise their impact simply by looking at these feelings square in the eye.

And when Great Aunt Sally plunges into another gaff, and when you find yourselves faced with the expectations of others, just smile and say 'we are trying'. One in four couples who are trying to conceive have fertility issues. You are so VERY NOT ALONE in this, so please do not feel this is a shameful secret.

And when your best friend needs to tell you her news and she is so afraid of how much it is going to hurt you, feel free to burst into tears together – she's your best friend! You can cry happiness for her, and cry sadness for yourself, and in every way the emotions in your heart will have an outlet. In being true to your feelings, you will resonate in a better place; maybe not great, but better. Being sad alone is twice as sorrowful, and being in sadness with a friend will always halve the burden.

Don't be afraid to tell others that you are struggling. You'll be amazed by the amount of love and support that pours towards you, by the empathy that will flow, for being truthful about your feelings will always help, no matter how hard it is. The people who love you will always want to help, and even if the things they say are sometimes not always the right thing, in accepting their well-meaning love and sympathy you will find strength in their support.

The biological clock

Many women do not meet the right man in their twenties, and you may find yourself looking down the powder keg that is the ticking of that dreaded biological clock. Tick-tock. Everyday you feel like the inexorable passing of time is washing your fertility away.

First, let me reassure you that the clock is simply a biological factor driven through your DNA, it is not something you can choose. The feelings of needing to have a child are inherent in our humanness and most of us are hardwired to feel this. The wish to get pregnant is not something we can turn on and off like a tap, it just is.

Every one of us is born with the need to propagate the species, we are programmed to want to have babies. Granted, there is a small percentage of the population who choose not to (apparently it is 5 per cent – who figures this stuff out?!).

The thing about trying to conceive for the first time in our thirties and forties is that biologically it is more of a challenge for us. And that is OK. So long as you are able to look at that challenge in a realistic light, then you have every chance of helping nature to do her job. Keeping in mind that even when we are walking down the assisted track, it is still very much about enabling the processes of nature.

Let us use the analogy of a marathon. If you were told tomorrow that you would be running the London Marathon, you would not expect to get off your couch and hey presto just get out there and run 26 miles! Hell no, you would need to start training, looking at all the ways that you could prepare your body for the task, building up day by day, week by week, month by month, improving your fitness, eating the right kinds of foods, thinking about your rest and exercise in the context of being fit enough to run such a long distance.

When we come to fertility, we need to apply the same mentality of preparation, applying everything that will help to bring us into shape for conception, gestation, birth and parenthood. So, if you find yourself challenged by the idea that the clock is ticking, rather than clenching into a paroxysm of denial and fear, think marathon, and start getting yourself in shape for going the distance.

As long as we are producing eggs, we have the opportunity to conceive. Doing all that we can do to enhance our egg and sperm quality (good nutrition) and by looking at all the lifestyle factors that enhance our health and vitality, we are investing ourselves in building and enhancing our sexual/conception energy. We are preparing ourselves to go the distance. And no one ever said that running 26 gruelling, slogging, sweaty miles was easy!

Everything you do in trying to conceive is preparing you mentally and physically for the challenges of parenthood. Stretch your minds and recognise the 26 miles in front of you will last until that child is 18 and beyond, so boy do you want to be in good shape!

Reproductive timeline – particular considerations for over-35s

So what is the biology of all this? And why do things shift at around the 35 mark?

In this section we are discussing age-related reproductive capacity primarily in female terms, although, saying that, all the factors of ageing do also affect men. Male reproduction is determined by hormone balances, not in the monthly cyclical way that women's reproduction is, and there are age-related shifts for men too.

The biggest male hormonal transition happens around their mid-forties, round about the moment they feel that running away in the little red convertible sports car with the leggy blonde bombshell model on board seems a really good idea. Don't worry, it's just a phase. There is a big testosterone surge at this time of life, just before his hormones go on the long, steady descent of lessening testosterone, hence lessening of his fertility.

It is just as important for men in their mid-thirties to make compensations for the toll that modern life exerts, given that 40 per cent of infertility issues are now male factor. Chronic stress and poor diet with insufficient quality of rest will affect male hormone balances. Sperm are hugely susceptible to the degradations of poor lifestyle and diet, so men in this age group of 35+ need to take really good care of their swimmers.

Both males and females are in their most vibrant fertility around 16–24, just when we are being told to take every precaution to *not* get pregnant. This astonishingly fertile vitality is a partly why teenage pregnancy rates are so high – well, that combined with the dire alcohol culture that is normal for most teenagers now (too many pregnancies occur under the influence).

Recently, a whole community of *Homo sapien* bodies from 30 000 years ago were discovered in a cave, and scientists were absolutely amazed to discover that their physiology was more or less identical to how we are now. This is interesting in the context of how our fertility is driven, because at that time the average life expectancy was around 30. So our peak of fertility of 24 meant that a child of 6 would stand every chance of surviving as part of the community without their parents. All these millennia later, our biological drive still reflects this.

As our life expectancy has elongated, so too has our peak fertility. Recent studies have shown that women are now in the fullness of their fertility until 28 or 29. Here is where we need to appreciate the reality of how fertility begins to change, for there is no crash, it just gradually diminishes. The denouement towards menopause is a long, slow, gentle slope towards 51–54, the average age of menopause here in the UK.

Between 28 and 35 there is a very slow incremental marginal shift towards a lessening of fertility in women. This is where the relationship between maternal age and egg quality *begins* to matter. This is different for every woman, and is entirely dependent on the combination of her genetic inheritance and the lifestyle that she has led. Does she come from a family with vibrant fertility? Is there a history of easy and prolific births? Any late pregnancies in the family? She must also look back to her puberty, and to her sexual and contraceptive choices, and ask if her lifestyle has affected the quality of her eggs.

The good news is that it is fairly easy to offset the taxations that lifestyle may have imposed in the past. As soon as we turn our hearts and minds to nourishing our fertility, we begin to enhance our fertile capacities.

In terms of biology and physiology, things do take a shift after 35. From 35–42, our fertility is beginning to decline, and it is more important to really pay attention. Some women will have an inherent fertility and not have too much difficulty conceiving, whereas others will need to work towards being birth-fit.

Birth-fit? But I thought we were talking about conception?

Well yes, we are. But the difference with the 35+ bracket is that having our first child in this stage of life is much more physiologically challenging. We must understand that 35-year-old sinews do not ease open in quite the way that 24-year-old sinews do, nor do they spring back again with quite the same ease! The nutritive balance in our body is what nourishes the bones, cartilage, sinews, ligaments, the muscles; *every* single tissue, every cell, very ovum, every sperm, is nourished by the foods and fluids we choose.

This is why good nutrition is *the* fundamental message for increasing our fertile capacities – it makes us more birth-fit.

It is interesting that Western medicine finds this significant shifting point at age 35. In Chinese medicine we understand the ages of development to run in 7-year cycles for women, and in 8-year cycles for men. By 14 the menstruation arrives, and throughout the phases to 21 and on to 28 we are in our peak fertility, at 35 we transition down from our most fertile time, at 42 we begin to shift towards the peri-menopause and at 49 we enter the menopause phase. Both Chinese and Western medicine acknowledge the timing of these shifts, as this is the biological reality of women's bodies.

I absolutely reiterate: every woman is different, and every woman is capable of producing a fertile egg right up until her very last period. In biological terms, the older we are, the older our eggs are. We are born with the number of eggs we will ever have, thus they are as old as we are. The margins of success do significantly decrease as we age, but, in the wise words of fertility expert Emma Cannon, 'expect a miracle'.

When we look at successful fertility later in life, we need to recognise that there is a fortuitous happenstance when the vital egg meets the vital sperm and there is a vital pregnancy, even into our late forties. This has happened to women throughout the ages. Late in life pregnancy is relatively uncommon, but it is not unusual.

This is why the advice in this book is so directed towards the importance of the replenishments. The more we build our nutrition, which means the nutrition of our sexuality, the nutrition of our mind/heart (happy thoughts) as much as the dietary and lifestyle changes, then the more we enhance our fertility. So when we are trying to conceive in this more mature age bracket, our emphasis must be all about quality.

Quality food, quality rest, quality work time, quality play time, and plenty of quality sex!

The myth of the cliff

Many women who are trying to conceive in their mid-thirties spend a great deal of time fearing the dreaded *forty* (said in a shake-the-rafters booming voice).

When we are talking about women trying to conceive, especially for the first time, there is this overwhelming idea that somehow 40 is a *cut off point*. But, you cannot go to bed age 39 and 364 days, and wake up the next morning with greatly reduced fertility, that's just not biology!

The myth of this number is primarily driven through the fact that, here in the UK, there must be guidelines as to how IVF is administered through the processes of the NHS and the spending of public monies on this kind of elective health care.

With biological logic, it has been determined that 40 is the cut off point within the NHS parameters. I am not arguing against the logic of why HFEA and the NHS have determined this number as the guideline, but it *is* logically arbitrary number across the *spectrum* of when a woman's fertility begins to decline. In fact, a woman's unique fertility profile will be significantly driven by the combination of her genetic inheritance, the overall quality of her diet and lifestyle, and her emotional status. When you are trying to conceive in this 35+ bracket it is vitally important that you set your heart and mind towards enhancing the fertility that you do have. For sperm *and* egg, no matter how old you are, you can still improve your fertile capacities.

A part of your fertility is the ability to have a fertile mind and a fertile heart, and a fertile relationship, living a fertile life filled with ideas and activities that interest you and engage you and connect you to being fully the person you are.

Please be assured that bringing yourself into optimum fertility *will* make you stronger and much more able to cope if a biological child is not on the cards for you.

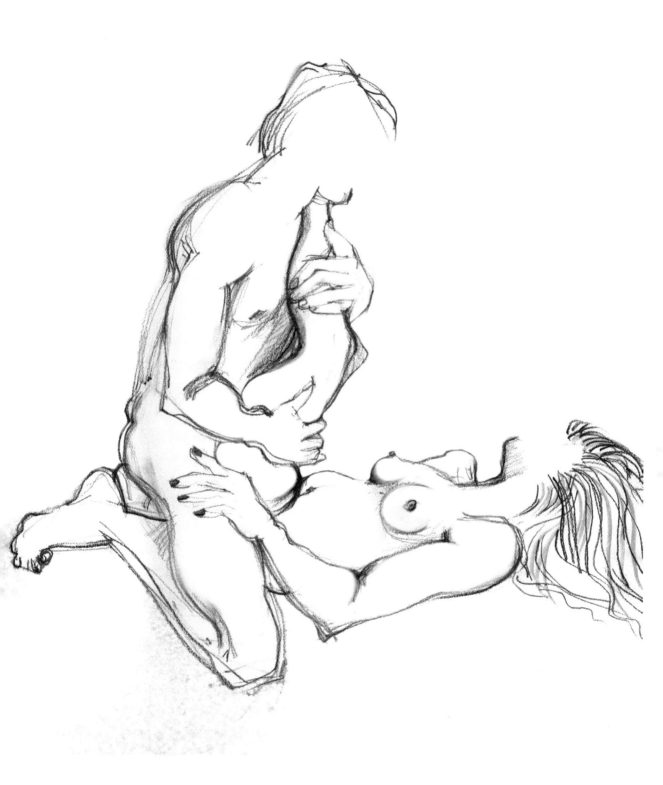

plunging

you delve
into the secret places
deep within me

sinking
you follow the perfume of my longing
your nose gently parting the fissure of my yearning
dropping within
to breathe deep of the scent of me
as my lips part with the slickness of my seeping juices
their heat touching your senses
with the need to plunge

with all of you
open wide
to encompass me
lips on lips
sliding
drawing
into the fall
to be filled with the thrusting of your tongue

plunging
into softness dreamt of
the shaking ripple of my need
clasping around your tongue
as it flickers a dance of delight upon my senses

for whirl this does take me
into a spiral of enchantment
cascading upward
a dizzy ascent to requirement
to be in the place you need me to be

thrusting, i writhe
altering, gyrating
swaying, diving
to find the place you most want to be
waiting
with baited breath
for the feeling of knowing
this
this is what you want

the exact place
where your plunge feels the way your shaft is in me
the driving hard lunge
of every millimetre of you
so thoroughly encompassed in me
that there is no true sense
of who is who
of where you begin, of where i end
just one
driving pure sensation
without beginning or end

and the purity of this fusion opens you further
to unleash
your Alpha
the part inside you
that wants to take without asking

and with fierceness you
rise to drive
the length of you
sheathed in the perfect welcome
that your tongue has danced upon me

the wanting in me
is as fierce as your desire

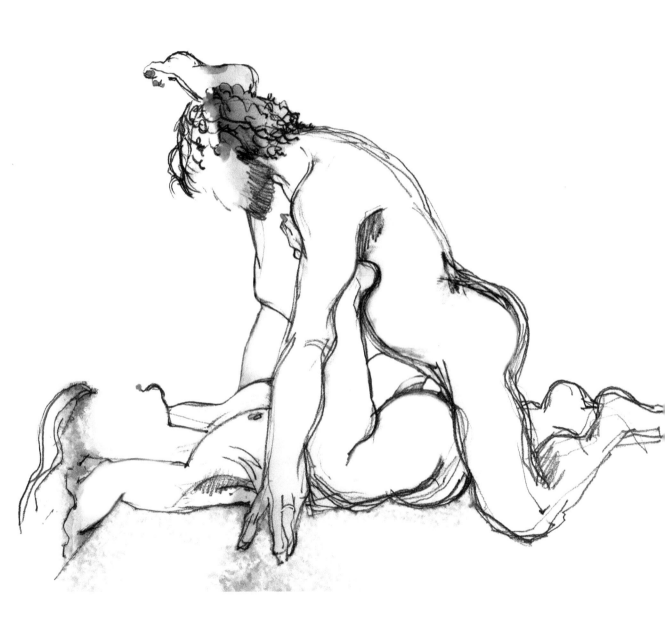

Chapter Fourteen

AMH and ovarian reserve – what does it really mean?

Testing for the levels of AMH (anti-mullerian hormone) is a method for determining ovarian reserve (the capacity of the ovary to provide eggs that are capable of being fertilised), via a blood test. For many years the standard evaluation of ovarian reserve was assessed through 'antral follicle count' whereby, under ultrasound, the numbers of antral follicles were counted. The FSH (follicle-stimulating hormone) and LH (luteinising hormone) levels were also assessed. This determined if a woman's follicle and hormone levels were a reflection of the appropriate numbers for her age.

In the last 10 years or so there have been significant studies to evaluate the results of measuring the AMH, and this blood test is now considered as a much superior way of evaluating women in the older age range as good candidates for IVF.

What this means is that AMH testing is being used to help assess if it is worthwhile to take a woman through a stimulation cycle, trying to determine if she will produce any eggs. In current fertility practice, the measurement of AMH is fast becoming a standard test for women who are struggling to conceive, and is now often used with younger women with unexplained infertility.

There is some emerging evidence that AMH levels can be influenced by race, body mass index and polycystic ovaries. It is becoming increasingly common for fertility units to use AMH testing as part of their standardised front line evaluation.

AMH markers help predict if a woman may be a candidate for ovarian hyper-stimulation, and may be an effective tool to determine if a woman may be at risk of ovarian hyper-stimulation syndrome (OHSS); if so, her drugs may be modified accordingly.

Worldwide, there is no agreed 'normal' level of AMH yet determined by the fertility experts. Different units use different measures, and results will vary from lab to lab, and from country to country. For example, a recent study showed that AMH measurements may be less accurate if the person being measured is vitamin D deficient.

What concerns us here is what can happen when a couple are told that the AMH is too low. When women are given the opportunity to Google this information, they very often jump to the conclusion that this is some kind of death knell to their chances of conceiving.

So, take a deep breath and let's not jump to the conclusion that this equates to an early menopause. Statistics vary greatly as to the rates of early menopause, from between 1–4 per cent, to 10 per cent, though most references suggest it is on average about 5 per cent. So if we consider that less than 5–10 per cent of women will be having a genuine early menopause, it is important to keep your hat on, not panic and figure out how this sliding scale of fertility markers relates to your personal biology.

AMH levels ought to be considered within the context of the LH (luteinising hormone) and FSH (follicle-stimulating hormone) levels (measured on day 1–3 of the menstrual cycle), and how your period behaves. For example, is your period regular? Is the flow straightforward with good volume, and no associated PMS symptoms? Is it an appropriate length, and are the follicular and luteal phases balanced? Is the temperature charting in the usual ranges? Does the progesterone level indicate regular ovulations?

If all these factors are in place it may be too soon to assume that this is a case of early menopause. Equally, if the AMH is low and the periods are erratic, maybe with a long follicular phase, then it is important to recognise that there is an ovulatory issue going on, and that this may indicate a low ovarian reserve.

Cancer treatments, tamoxifen (hormonal therapy for breast cancer), surgeries that may affect blood flow to the ovaries, auto-immune disorders, and chromosomal irregularities (Fragile X, Turner syndrome) can all influence early menopause.

Family history is very important too. Is there early menopause in the family? Especially your mother? Sister? Aunties? Grandmother? There is also a paternal link that can influence premature ovarian failure through transmission of the Fragile X chromosomal irregularity. Polycycstic Ovarian Syndrome relates to Metabolic Syndrome (sometimes called Syndrome X), which is more often inherited through the paternal genes.

Your family history is an important part of learning to understand your own unique profile, of which the AMH is one small part.

To panic, or not to panic

The most important thing to remember when coping with the news of low AMH is that although it does indicate a fertility issue, it is not a definitive statement that you are infertile.

The best thing to do is to work with your gynaecologist or fertility consultant to consider exactly what your personal profile is, within the context of the AMH blood result. It may be a very helpful indicator that IVF is a good track for you, or that it is not, saving you all the physical and financial stresses of the intervention.

In Chinese medicine terms the emphasis would be to turn our attention to the eggs that you do have, to work to regulate the cycle, to help enhance the capacity that may be there to help ovulate a viable egg. This is where our approach of pre-conception care is so important. We look at the biology of folliculogenesis (the maturation of the ovarian follicle) to help develop the potential from the eggs that are there and the TCM advice is 4–6 months of regular herbal treatment coupled with a focused attention to diet and lifestyle.

Rather than wallowing in a sense of hopelessness and despair, it is vital for you to turn your attention to all that you can do to increase your chances of producing viable eggs. Find the ways to care for yourself and each other with loving attention and tons of oxytocin to keep yourselves in that parasympathetic place, to work together to tackle the lifestyle changes that can influence your health on every level.

Many people will have been given the news that the AMH is low right at the beginning of their fertility investigations, and it may be that you haven't yet taken on board all the considerations that are the constant theme of this book. The testing that is being done to investigate why you have not conceived is looking at a handful of hormonal markers. While those test results are a reflection of your health, your hormonal balance can always be influenced by improving your diet and lifestyle.

AMH is a protein, not an actual hormone. The amount of the AMH protein that is being measured is influenced by the way that your digestive and reproductive hormones are working, or not. If your AMH is being done following a very stressful time – bereavement, relationship crisis, work-related difficulties, moving house – then the readings may be influenced by the fact that you have been in a chronic sympathetic state.

Our follicles are released on a 150-day cycle and the AMH reading is being taken from the follicles that have already been initiated within that 150 days. This is why our Chinese medicine advice is to give the diet and lifestyle changes, acupuncture and herbs a full 4–6 months to help influence better fertility, potentially increasing better activation of healthy follicles.

If you are feeling uncertain about what you are being told, and perhaps you are not comfortable with the way you are being told (some couples find the information can be given in a rather 'wham bam thank you ma'am' sort of way), please express your confusion and be sure to ask for the fullest clarification.

Do not hesitate to ask for further testing of your other biological markers and chromosomal markers, to have as much information as possible to help evaluate what your AMH levels may mean in the overall context of your fertility.

AMH is not a single defining factor, it is one part of the total picture of your whole unique and individual biology.

Folliculogenesis

So now let us look a little further into the biology of reproduction.

Folliculogenesis describes the process by which the woman's primordial follicles are brought forward into the cycle that is her ovulation and menstruation, potential conception and pregnancy. (The primordial follicles consist of the ovum – egg – enclosed in a single layer of cells, the follicle.)

Primordial follicles are the microscopic follicles that you are born with. In folliculogenisis (literally 'follicle' and 'beginning') the first thing that happens is called initiation, whereby the primordial follicle is activated. This initiated follicle is then brought forward into the development process, first coming through a primary and secondary phase, to develop forward to the pre-antral then early antral phase. At this stage the follicles are minuscule, between 0.2 and 0.4 mm, and the whole process takes about 65 days.

As these early antral follicles are being processed, the viable (ones likely to hold a quality egg) follicles move forward to becoming antral follicles, developing up to 2 mm in size. These are the follicles that can be measured via the antral follicle counting done by an ultrasound scan. These antral stage follicles are the ones from which the AMH is measured.

During the initiation of the primordial follicle and the development to the antral stage (about 90 days), there is a simultaneous process going on called atresia. Of all the follicles that have been initiated, a certain number of them will be non-viable. These are sent into a state of atresia, which means that they stop developing.

After 3 months, the antral follicles that have reached 2 mm are now the cache of follicles that will be brought forward for the processes towards ovulation. The next phase is called selection, and as the antral follicles grow towards 5 mm, the non-viable follicles are moved into atresia while the viable follicles are ready and waiting for the next level of development. This is when the body selects the most likely follicles for the next, most important, part of the process.

The next phase is the maturation stage, now 140 days from the point of initiation. This coincides to the day when your period comes. On day 1 of your cycle, as the FSH and LH hit the cache of selected follicles, usually about 4 or 5 follicles will pick up the stimulation from the FSH and begin to develop. It's a bit of a race, and only one will become the dominant follicle. Only the most viable one of the selected follicles will be the one to take over, to grasp all of the available FSH and LH, to be the one to ovulate.

Can you see how clever nature is? All through this process of folliculogenesis the body is constantly sifting and sorting, sending to atresia the non-viable follicles, and bringing forward the follicles that contain the healthiest eggs, and then given the handful of likely contenders, bringing forward the most viable. Like the acorn that may one day become a mighty oak, inside that egg is the map of another whole person, a package of DNA that is filled with all the tendencies and reactions of the person they will become – well, half of the potential person anyway. The other half is in that viable sperm, the one that is the strongest swimmer with the mightiest energy to pierce that egg and begin the melding.

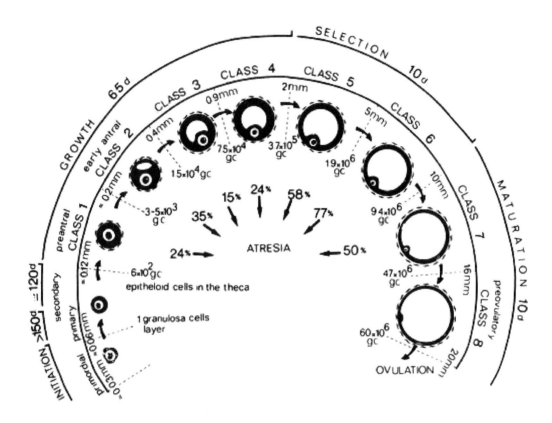

From Human Reproduction 1986 Feb; 1(2):81–7. Dynamics of follicular growth in the human: a model from preliminary results. Gougeon, A. Reproduced with permission.

I never tire of talking about this, for every time that I do, I am struck again with awe by the absolute eloquence of nature's ways. And I very much hope that I have conveyed how vital preconception care is. The nutrition we input into our bodies is the very thing that is nourishing the follicles and sperms as they develop. If there aren't enough good nutrients during these processes of folliculogenesis and spermatogenesis (the process in which spermatozoa are produced), this will affect the health of those sperms and eggs.

We need really good nutrition to affect the calibre of the development, selection and maturation of the follicles and the spermatazoa. And, by staying in parasympathetic response we help our body to have a fluent HPO – hypothalamus, pituitary, ovarian (gonadal) axis. This hormone feedback loop helps to govern the smooth and effective process of the sperm and egg maturation.

The more normalised our hormone balance is, the better these processes can occur. Bang-bang-bang (she beats her drum standing on a soapbox shouting loudly – *nutrition is vital!*); daily life can beat the crap out of our smooth functioning, and chronic stress and/or switchy stress responses interrupt our hormonal sequencing.

Good food, Good loving, Good rest. This is the Good recipe for making Good babies.

When the egg and sperm quality is too low ... to donor or not to donor?

Before we leave this discussion in respect of the quality of gametes (egg and sperm) it is important to drop in a word about donor eggs, sperm or embryos.

In recent years this has become a very strong trend within assisted conception. Many couples choose to go to other countries, many of the fertility units in the UK provide joint support with these overseas and European donor facilities. There is an increasing provision for donor options at the UK units, and we are now seeing the emergence of donor agencies here in the UK.

In many of the fertility units the words 'low AMH' and 'donor' will be used in the same sentence, and very often the advice from the fertility consultants will be to go straight to donor IVF.

The units should provide you with a counselling service prior to making this choice, and it is very important for you to fully consider what the donor route may mean for your emotional well-being.

Many couples have landed in my office feeling a bit lost and confused and not at all clear about what it may mean to parent a donor child. As a completely personal observation, I would suggest that some units provide a somewhat cursory approach to counselling parents regarding the fullest ramifications of parenting a donor child, and I would encourage you to thoroughly explore the issues around the donor option before making this important choice. You may find that the counselling services offered by the fertility units will emphasise the statistics, and that the counselling will be more focused on managing a donor IVF cycle.

To be very clear, I fully respect that the fertility units are focused on helping you to find a pathway to conceive a child, and I offer these observations in light of my training in the broader spectrum of total care that comes with Chinese medicine.

Going down the donor road is not just about getting pregnant, it is also about really exploring what it will mean to have a child. With sperm and egg donation there is the surety that 50 per cent of that baby's DNA will belong to one of you; with donor embryo you will be birthing a child who is not genetically connected to either of you.

I encourage you to explore something called 'genetic bewilderment'. This is a psychological condition now recognised by both the American Psychological Association and British Psychology Society, and it is all about what adopted and donor children may experience in respect of having a 'knowing' inside of them that is their genetic tendency, and the fact that they do not see and feel these 'knowings' in their family.

This can trigger a feeling of bewilderment in both the child and the parents. Children learn through imitation, and when our traits fully match there is a sense of belonging. When there are traits that are not reflected back at us, this can lead to this sense of bewilderment. This is especially important to bear in mind when making the choice to have a donor embryo.

In America, a donor embryo is referred to as 'in-utero adoption'. I believe this is a very helpful term, for it gives you the perspective that is so important when making this choice. I truly believe that one should make this choice following the sort of counselling given to couples who choose to adopt.

In respect of choosing either donor sperm or donor egg, it is vital for you both to fully unpack the potential for jealousy, uncertainty and resentment. It is important to explore the potentially negative sides of this decision, as well as the potential joys of having a child together.

In all my years of supporting couples I have seen countless happy families and many wonderful bonds between happy, centred, secure children and their non-biological parents. For many couples this has been a marvellous way for them to step into parenthood. Creating a delightful space and place for these children to grow up in, loved and treasured by aware parents who allow them to step fully into who they actually are within the context of their own genetic load is a gift for everyone: for the parents, for the children and for all the extended family and friends.

Please be mindful not to rush this decision, and remember that you will be raising this child through all their stages of growth and into their adulthood. This is about so much more than just getting pregnant. A certified fertility practitioner will have access to the most recent literature and should be able to help you into a fulsome understanding of all that donor entails.

Surrogacy

Here in the UK we have an excellent not-for-profit organisation called Surrogacy UK that offers information and support and gives access to a whole community of advice and care and quality guidance (see the Useful Resources).

Surrogacy is a very important option for couples who may not be able to have a biological child together, and should your resources deem this a viable option I encourage you to explore guidance from a well-qualified source.

Every child is a gift, no matter how they land up in our lives, and it is one of the great good fortunes of our modern society that so many options are now accessible and accepted.

Find the solutions that work for you.

Plan B

One of the important aspects of your journey to conceive a biological child – by whatever combination of his, hers, or donor – is to hold a space in your hearts to recognise that this may not happen for you.

As terrible as this thought might be, it is much healthier for you both to recognise that this may be a possibility.

This does not mean that you cannot still fully and completely *dare to hope*, for this will always be the very thing that opens you to the fullness of your receptivity.

Considering your plan B opens up a space within your relationship to explore what it really means for each of you to become parents together, and to factor how you each may feel about adoption, or fostering. There are so very many children out there who are just as desperate in their desire to have a mother and father as you may feel about having a child.

I urge you to take the time to explore together how you may feel should there not be a conception between you.

Should you find that having a child in your lives is more important than whether or not there is a biological conception, it may be helpful to explore your adoption options, either through the NHS or through private agencies, or to consider if fostering may be a way for you to share your lives with a child.

These processes can take some time so may be helpful to explore in advance, perhaps to get on to any waiting lists, and to determine what the eligibility and vetting processes may entail.

The Infertility Network, INUK, have a website called More to Life (*www.infertilitynetworkuk.com/moretolife/*), an excellent resource and support network.

Reaching out for support can be a great help to embrace the fortitude to cope with such a disappointment, and to develop whatever else you may wish to welcome into your lives. If the privilege of a biological child is not going to happen for you, it is important to recognise what else can use your parenting energies – fostering a business into fruition, expanding your career, taking the opportunity to change careers, doing a degree in something you feel passionate about, fostering your creative self making art, writing, perhaps making music …

Plan B should be something that sings to your heart and fosters your passion.

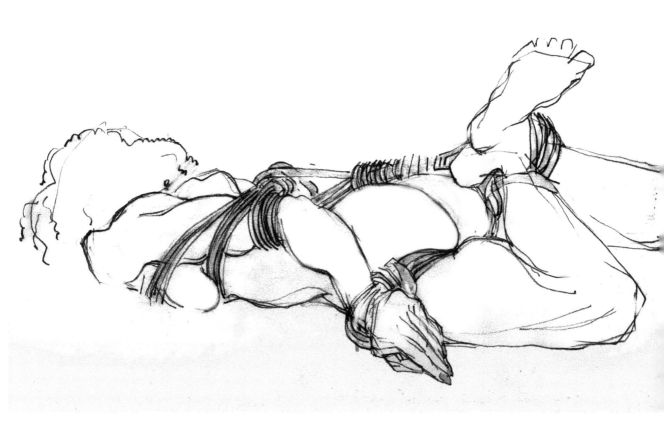

push

i love to be pushed
i love to be restrained

tie me up to set me loose
consummate liberty

with very knot further unbound
dropping into wild
abandoned, unravelled
unfurl me with each twist and turn
opening wider as all closes in

the push of force
subtle control
held by will, nothing more
elegance in such dominion

relinquishment into capitulation

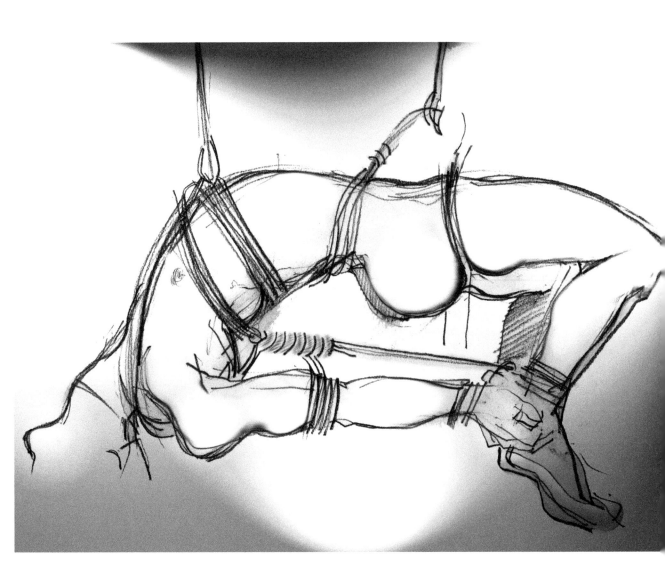

Chapter Fifteen

Making IVF fun – well – in the very least OK ...

What?!

How can IVF be *fun*??

OK, maybe fun is not necessarily the best word to choose, but IVF does not need to be horrible, and it most certainly does not need to be stressful.

Pardon?!

I can confirm that IVF does not need to be at all stressful. Granted it is filled with a dash of excitement tempered with a dose of trepidation, coupled with the amplified feeling of being on that roller coaster of hope and fear.

When IVF came into prominence in the eighties it was indeed very stressful. The units were still learning how to help manage people's experience of the process. Every unit did things their own way, and on top of it all, most people did not talk about the fact that they were undergoing fertility treatment.

In those early days, pre-IVF being available on the NHS, a greater portion of the people who were undergoing treatment were in higher stress jobs in higher income brackets. Then, because there were a relatively large proportion of media people having IVF, many of them chose to write articles and books about their experiences. They began to talk about IVF in magazines, on chat shows.

What this generated was an impression of how difficult and stressful the whole experience could be, which back then it most certainly was. It was this significant discussion in both the regular and social media that normalised the IVF experience, alongside the Internet's information base. Then the UK government decided that IVF would be made available on the NHS, and the huge seed change occurred that has really revolutionised the processes, as now a great many more people can access this kind of fertility treatment, regardless of their income. And over these ensuing years there has been an accompanying *vast* improvement in how the units prepare and manage clients for the processes of IVF.

Nowadays every unit will host open evenings, where they offer couples a step-by-step presentation about the processes, with a chance to listen first hand to the consultants, nurses and embryologists, to help couples determine if this is the right unit for them.

If you are paying privately, I always urge couples to go to several different units' open evenings and to consider how the location of the unit works in relation to their work-home-unit triangle. It is really important to try and assess the path of least resistance.

Within the NHS system you be allocated to the unit that your PCT (Primary Care Trust) has contracted, so you will not have a choice about which unit you will attend.

It is important to organise your diaries to allow for the time to make sure that you can easily manage the travel logistics that might be involved.

Units will give you a sequence of dates for your meds and scans and blood tests, all of which is a slightly moveable feast, depending on how you respond, but does give you a good outline from which to plan your schedule for your IVF weeks.

Many people are genuinely surprised when they realise that there is not actually too much running around involved. On the standard long protocol (course of IVF) you will start sniffing IVF drugs in the form of nasal spray on day 21 of your cycle, then your next appointment is 3 weeks later for your blood test. During a follow-up phone call you are instructed when to start your stimulation drugs, then there are usually 2 check visits for scans and bloods to assess the follicle development and to check your womb lining. Pending what they find, there may be another scan or blood test, then collection, then transfer. Over the 6 weeks of the managed aspect of your IVF, you are really only in the unit a handful of times.

Caveat: there are a few units in London that maintain a very much higher rate of monitoring, so this is a question to take with you to the open evenings.

Most of the units now use a patient number tracking system, allowing whoever answers the phone to bring your file up on their screen, so now much of the communication can be managed via phone calls.

As I've said, the units have become highly adept at making the timings and systems very straightforward for couples. What is smart thinking is to draw a line around the 6–8 weeks of your IVF cycle and ensure that your diary minimises other commitments during this time so that you are free to focus on taking really good care of each other during these weeks.

During your IVF it is vitally important for you to maintain a maximum of oxytocin-inducing contact and loving touch. By putting that level of physical intimacy into your IVF, you will most certainly help to enhance your fertile Fizz. Loving is way more fun than stressing so I'm all for making IVF more fun.

IVF and sexuality – lovemaking and burgeoning ovaries

Let's figure it out. Women ovulate only one dominant follicle from one ovary each month, alternating each month, meaning that the opposite ovary is ovulating every 8 weeks.

During the IVF process, any number of follicles are stimulated up to dominant size on both ovaries simultaneously. That's a serious amount of action happening all at once, which is why the IVF stimulation phase was originally dubbed 'super-ovulation'.

This means that there will be a excess fluid and inflammation within the pelvic cavity, loads of fluids sent into the region to buffer and protect the ovaries, and this is why mild OHSS (ovarian hyper-stimulation syndrome) is a normal part of about 33 per cent of IVFs. Most women will not be feeling enormously sexual with that amount of tender activity going on!

My advice that this is a time for gentle non-penetrative sensual tenderness. Likewise, the down-regulation phase is a time when the hormone treatment is influencing the HPO to shut down, ergo, the oestrogen complexes are being switched off. These are the hormones that help to drive our sexual desire, so often there is not enough oestrogen driven oomph to recommend sexual activity during this time. Most women will not feel very sexy without those HPO drivers of LH and FSH to pump up the oestrogen.

Down-regulation sets the body into a false menopause, halting the ovulatory function. This is why the menopausal symptoms of emotional lability (bitchiness, tearfulness, irritability), and hot flushes and headaches are a relatively normal set of symptoms during this phase. The way a woman experiences her 'down-reg' will be hugely influenced by her pre-existing condition, and the way her symptoms will develop during the down-reg will most certainly relate to her pre-IVF hormonal status.

The IVF protocols are a time to focus on loving support. I cannot emphasise enough how important it is to bring your attention to cherishing each other in a less sexual manner. Add to the switching off of the hormone cascades, and the tensions of anticipation, fear and worry, and you may have a recipe for sympathetic dominance.

By focusing on the loving touch that helps to keep us in parasympathetic you will go miles towards helping engender the Fizz that is such a vital part of the conception process. Kisses, cuddles, hand-holding, naked full body contact are all the ways that we can draw up the oxytocin without needing to be in the throes of sexual bliss. By all means if genuine randiness is there, go for it. But in all honesty, it's not likely.

Girls, 6 weeks is a long time to not have penetrative sex, and with a positive pregnancy it could end up being rather longer if you are feeling too delicate in the first trimester to think about lovemaking. Do remember how important hand jobs and blow jobs are for keeping that sexual tension thrumming between you. There is nothing like an orgasm to bring on the oxytocin!

Guys, say thank you with a fat dose of pampering and reciprocate the sharing of oxytocin with lots of stroking, kissing and cuddling.

The key during the weeks of an IVF cycle, from the onset of down-reg, through the stim-phase to the transfer, and then through the treacle of the wait to the test day, is a time to focus on cherishment. This is a marvellous time to find all the ways that you can show your lover just how much they matter to you. I always suggest to couples that IVF is a perfect time to re-visit the initial romance of dating.

Distract yourselves with romantic dinners, go to the movies, walk in the park holding hands, re-connect to those early days when all you could think about was the next time you would see each other, exploring each other's thoughts and feelings, re-connecting to the thrill of discovering this person you are so attracted to.

The first flush of love is fraught with oxytocin, so allowing yourselves to sink back into the vibe of initial attraction is a sure-fire way to re-kindle the flows of oxytocin that are the ultimate bonding hormone.

IVF is a mindset. If you choose to experience it as a walking-on-egg-shells stressful time, then it will be. Equally, you can choose for it to be an opportunity to fall in love again, opening wide all the true-heart connection that has brought you together, and affirming the lovemaking that is always at the heart of conception.

Babies want to be with happy people.

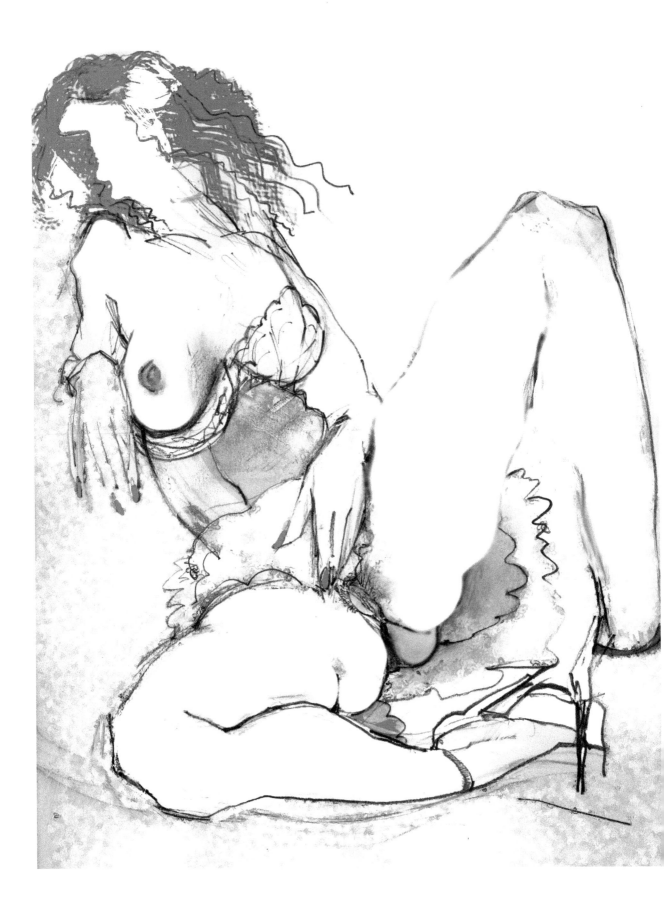

taste

memories, blink, gasp
clench, as i quiver with the remembered feel of you
inside me, thrumming
pumping, bursting

i love to feel you cum inside me
i feel so privileged to experience the naked you
i adore the way you orgasm
it makes me judder with a deep longing
to swallow you, whole
to milk you, to drink you

i love when you lap your cum from me
then moist and slippery, reach up to kiss me deep
the mingle of our tastes so sweet and bright
so musky and potent
i love the way we taste together upon each other's breaths

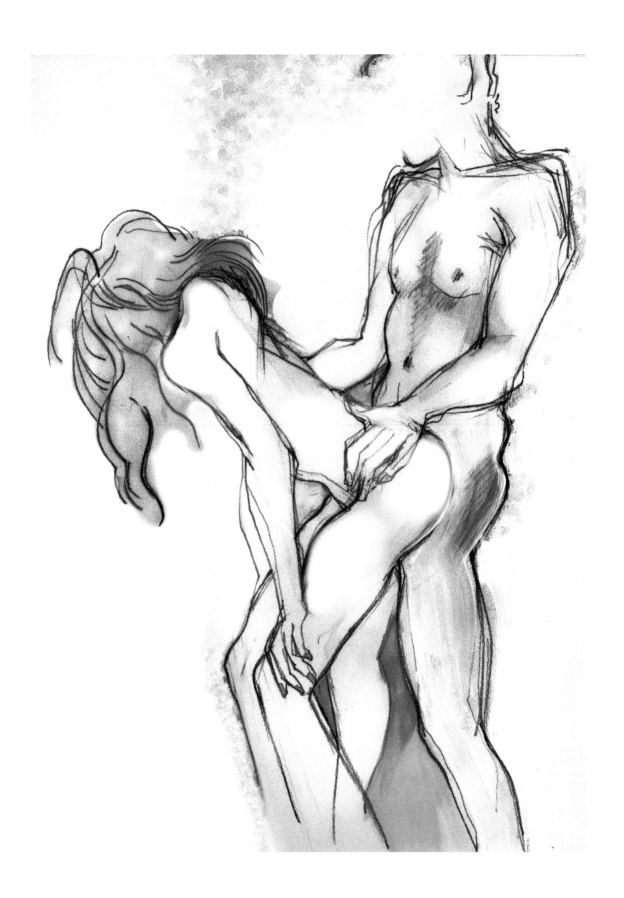

Chapter Sixteen

What is the correct diet for fertility?

Wow, giant question, just how long *is* a piece of string??

There are, without question, all the no-brainer factors of what *not* to eat, in respect of clearing your diet of any additives and preservatives, taking out refined foods, minding that you don't take caffeine and alcohol (except champagne of course!): in a nutshell, ensuring that you are not investing any toxic or non-food substances into the temple of your body.

In the sense that this book reflects the mantra 'you are what you think', it is also saying 'you are what you eat'.

When you are trying to conceive, it is important to always remember that the vitality and health of those sperm and ovum are directly determined by the quality of what you eat, the quality of the fluids your drink, the quality of the rest you take and the quality of any supplements you may need.

Rest is a very important nourishment, and being in bed by 11 p.m. can really help to set up your digestion for the morning, and improve the uptake capacities in your digestive systems that will help to improve your overall nutritional status.

You have an immense control over the health of your sperm and eggs (gametes), and when you are trying to conceive there is nothing quite as important as the nutrition you input. This is why good-quality nutritional supplements are so important, why Chinese herbs may bring a significant boost, why every bit of food you eat needs to be of the best value possible. This is why it is so important to eat as organically as you can.

On the organic note, my plea is to ensure that any animal products are as organic as possible. This is over and above buying organic fruit and veg. Commercial meat and dairy products are highly adulterated in respect of how the animals are husbanded (antibiotic overuse is a big issue) and slaughtered, so wherever possible please try to ensure your dairy and meat or meat products are organic. Farmed fish is highly adulterated, and I would recommend avoiding this wherever possible.

Everything that you invest into your body nourishes and influences the health of the sperms and eggs. Food is the first medicine, and through diet we have the strongest and most influential way to help our bodies into optimum health.

The most important message is wholefoods. If it is not a food in the complete state that nature intended, then please ask yourself if it is necessary for your body. Take, for example, margarine. We live in a world whereby there is an ingrained message that margarine is a healthier option than butter, a hangover from the message that saturated fats are bad for you.

Too many saturated fats are indeed not good for you, but saturated fats are still an important part of a healthy diet, and they are *essential* for your fertility. Hormones are lipophilic. Lipo = fats, philic = to love. This means that hormones rely on fat molecules to be transported around the body. So we *need* whole fats to have a healthy hormone balance.

Saturated fats *should* make up about 8 per cent of your daily diet, and the quality of those saturated fats is paramount. Organic butter is an excellent-quality wholefood saturated fat, but margarine is not a wholefood. Margarine is a trans fat, the process whereby an oil is hydrogenated in order to become a hard substance. There are many health risks associated to trans fats. Many of the margarines promote that they are low in saturated fat – the very thing we most need to carry those fertility hormones.

In Chinese medicine the subject of dietetics (the energy of food) has long been studied, and over many centuries the Chinese have determined the myriad ways that individual foods affect and nourish the body. Happily, I can report that butter is considered one of the best foods for Qi circulation, boosting the way that your energy is moving within. Butter, I would argue, is good for your libido.

And now you have just learned the secret to the success of my fertility practice. I am always telling people to eat butter, drink champagne and not go to the gym more than twice a week. Patients love my advice!

The point in this example is to outline that our digestion is well suited to draw nutrition from foods in their *whole* state, and that by turning your attention towards a diet which is about real food, you will greatly enhance your health and the health of your gametes (eggs or sperms).

If you found out you were pregnant tomorrow, you would not need to be persuaded to change your diet to only eating healthful foods. Well, pre-fertilisation, that sperm and that egg are that baby-to-be.

So my advice is to begin to make the changes in your eating habits right now, and then when you are pregnant you are already in the correct habit of wholefoods, clean foods, for the healthy development of your baby. And when that baby is born you will already be eating the right kind of diet for the best possible breast milk and recovery from childbirth, and by the time you are weaning you will be feeding your child on a healthful wholefood-orientated diet that will help them to grow fit and strong on healthy, happy vital foods.

It's a no-brainer! Make the changes now that you would expect to make for your child anyway.

Remember, those gametes may become that baby.

The importance of breakfast

'Eat breakfast like a king, lunch like a prince, and supper like a pauper.'
Health movement pioneer Adelle Davis (1904–74)

This is a most excellent saying and it is very attuned to the way our body is designed to work. I'm going to take us back to that Chinese medicine thing again, when we discussed circadian rhythms and I introduced you to the idea of the Chinese body clock. (Let us remember that the channel systems are all named for the organ they are associated to.)

According to this Chinese medicine clock, 7–9 a.m. are the Stomach hours, and 9–11 a.m. are the Spleen-pancreas hours. This is why we should breakfast like a king! The stomach does the digesting, and the spleen-pancreas has a fundamental influence on the uptake of the nutritional value within our food. Breakfast is the best time to be taking your nutritional supplements, so that the enhancement of nutritional input will be absorbed with the digestion of your food.

Breakfast is an important time for good-quality protein, and the continental style of having eggs, cheese and cold cuts in the morning meal is a great way to start the day. Digesting a protein will help to stabilise your blood sugar, especially if you are combining it with a low glycaemic index (GI) quality carbohydrate.

For many people, breakfast is often skipped in the dash to get off to work, and many find they do not have a good appetite in the morning. This is often because people are having their main meal in the evening, quite late. This taxes the digestion greatly, as these are the hours when the Stomach and Spleen-pancreas are least active. Not to mention that filling up on a heavy meal late at night is a disaster for your libido! If the stomach is busy digesting this will inhibit the free flow of your sexual hormones.

Skipping breakfast will often manifest as a coffee and muffin mid-morning type of start to the food day. This is a bit of a disaster for your blood sugar balance, offers little in the way of nutrition, taxes your system with the trans fats and additives factors that are rife in commercially baked goods (which are full of refined flour and refined sugar), the caffeine spikes the adrenals, and you end up on a roller coaster of digestive hormone upset that plays havoc with your energy, your libido, and your sperm and egg development ...

For many years I made sandwiches for my boys and for my husband. These were sandwiches for breakfast! Husband was a classic can't-eat-in-the-morning type, and the boys were ever on the dash to catch their bus in time.

Every morning I would send them off with 2 wholemeal pitta bread sandwiches, always with a protein filling and some kind of vegetable combo, lettuce, grated carrots, cucumber, salsa, pesto. They were under strict instructions to have one sandwich on the bus, so that they would arrive at school with their blood sugar in balance, ready and able to give better concentration to their work, and to have the other sandwich at mid-morning break, good-quality fuel to lead them up to lunch.

(Years later I learned that those sandwiches had the highest trading value at either of their schools, and they could exchange them for virtually anything from the other kids' tuck. Luckily, my boys usually wanted the sandwich over the junk.)

If you find it difficult to fit breakfast into your morning routine, just set your alarm for ten minutes earlier. The trick is to have all the ingredients ready in the fridge so that you can just lightly soften the pitta in the toaster, slap in the protein with the dressing of choice – mayo, salsa, horseradish, mustard, whatever taste sensation grabs your fancy – load it up with a handful of any veg combo and throw them in your bags, then as you sit through your morning commutes you both have a healthful breakfast to start your day on.

Lunch like a prince. Not so easy in most people's work environments. I recognise this can be a real challenge, and that it is very normal to eat a sandwich for lunch, often from a supermarket packet, full of trans fats, additives, stabilisers, preservatives, etc.

Many people eat in front of the computer and this is genuinely bad for your digestion. It is so important to take breaks away from the screen, to give your body a rest from the electromagnetic radiations, and it is healthful for your digestion to eat with focus and concentration, chewing well and allowing time to settle the food and absorb what you have eaten.

The trick is to look for recipes for a healthful and nutritious lunch, something that you can easily pack into take-away boxes and eat at room temperature, no need to heat up that will provide you with just the sort of nutrition that your body really needs. Batch cooking at the weekend is the best way to get into the routine of having this kind of nutritious food easily to hand in the busy working week. (I am in the process of writing 'The Take Your Lunch to Work Book' – so watch this space ...)

The objective here is to stoke up on strong and vital foods at the right times of day to ensure that you are bringing your body the right kind of sustaining fuel – balancing low GI happy gamete kind of foods.

Having loaded your prime nutrition into the early and mid part of the day then supper like a pauper is the right way to eat, as having a main meal late into the evening is not helpful for your digestive balance, or for your libido.

Changing your eating habits to these more physiologically appropriate eating patterns will greatly enhance your overall health, and this Fizzier approach to helping your hormone balance will go a very long way to improving your libido!

Insulin balance is vital for fertility

The endocrine of your digestion is fundamental to the balance of your sexual/conception hormones. Our HPO (hypothalamus, pituitary, ovarian (gonadal) axis) feedback loops, the balance of the FSH, LH, oestrogen, testosterone, progesterone, are all significantly influenced by the insulin levels in our blood.

You have no doubt heard people talk about insulin, usually in the context of words like hypoglycaemia (blood sugar levels are too low), hyperglycaemia (blood sugar levels are too high), insulin resistance, and, of course, diabetes. But many people do not really understand how insulin should work, or why a low glycaemic index (GI) is important, or even what glycaemic index actually is. In fact, our fertility hormones are dependent on our insulin levels being in balance.

This is one of the key reasons that I am always on about the importance of diet in fertility. It is not just about the nutritional input of what we eat, but it is also very much about the functionality of the foods we eat. When we eat highly refined foods, processed foods, a big part of the breakdown of that food has already been done – the bit that should actually be done by our bodies. Not only that, but what has been stripped out of the foods will often be what makes it more nutritious in the first place.

It is the process of breaking down the foods that is fundamental to the health of our metabolism. By asking our body to work with real foods, wholefoods, unrefined foods, we task our metabolism into the sort of workout that keeps it in great shape and good balance. When we fill our bodies with highly refined foods then it only does a fraction of that workout, and the metabolism does not function as well as it should.

Are you with me? This is why the wholefoods message is the foundation to genuinely healthy eating. Foods in a refined state have been stripped out, and the chemistry of the food is altered, thus when we go to digest that refined food, our bodies' chemistry is also altered away from the complex that it needs for optimum function.

Refined foods tend to have a higher glycaemic index, and foods which are in an unrefined state tend to have a lower GI. This is sometimes referred to as glycaemic load, and usually as GI. Glycaemic refers to 'glucose in the blood' = blood sugar.

The role of insulin in digestion is to metabolise the glucose in the body. Glucose is one of our main fuel sources. Insulin facilitates the conversion of the glucose into glycogen, which is then stored in the adipose tissues. This gives us a reserve of energy, as the body can then convert the glycogen back into a usable glucose when we need energy.

Low GI categorises foods that are complex carbohydrates or sugars that will require a significant level of breakdown in order to release and metabolise the glucose. These are referred to as 'slow carbs'. Low GI foods give us a more sustained stronger energy.

High GI means that much of this breakdown process is already done, usually via the refining process, so by time the carb reaches the digestive level there is not much work to do in order to convert the glucose, thus these are referred to as simple carbohydrates or 'fast carbs'. With fast carbs you will end up with higher levels of blood sugar at a much faster rate. This gives us a rather speedy spike of energy, and we will inevitably have a corresponding crash after the spike of the fast carb fuel is used up.

This generates unstable blood sugar levels. The glucose levels in the blood see-saw, and our metabolism swings from spike to crash.

But it gets a bit more complicated than just an in/out fuel source situation. When we ingest a high GI carb/sugar, the blood sugar spikes, and the pancreas releases a flood of insulin to deal with the flood of excess glucose. We end up with a great deal of excess insulin in the bloodstream.

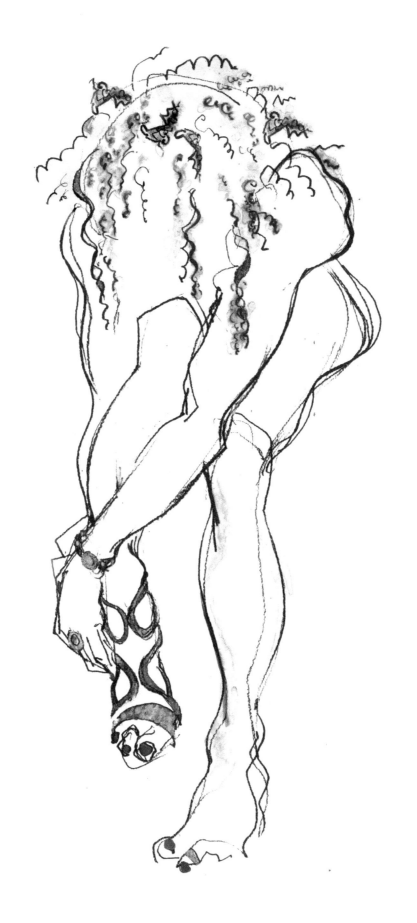

take me

i want to feel you take me to the places you want to go
such a simple creature am i
a harlot in my soul
a maiden at the mercy of the ravishing buccaneer
wanting nothing more than to be captive to a man's desires
desiring most monstrously to cast off the vanilla mantle of my everyday ladylike self
and to be melded to your wishes
stuff me, drive me, reel me, peel me
suck, fuck, lick, sip, sup and ply me
within every aperture you can find
and all the while there is but one thing i most want
my greatest reward is when you let me suck you
for feeling your cock in my mouth
is perhaps how I can show you how I feel

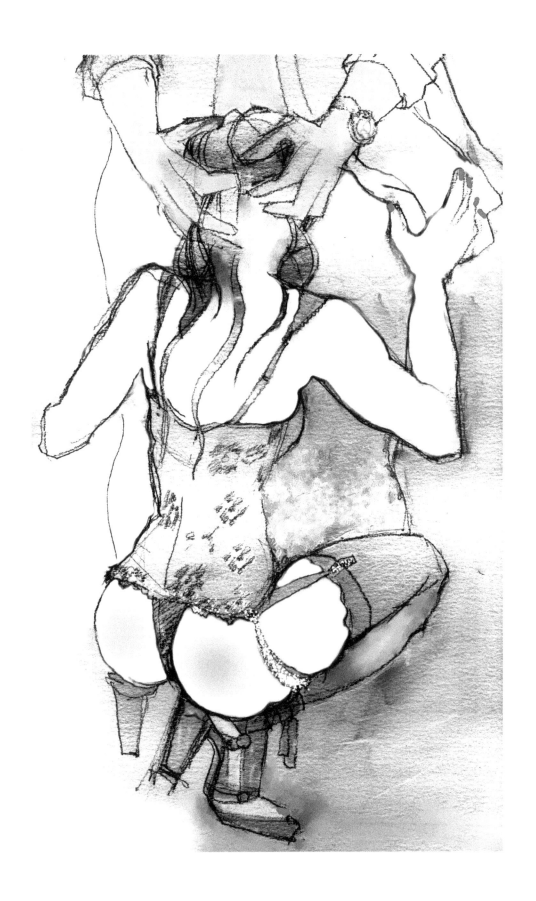

Chapter Seventeen

Insulin resistance

Across the Western world we have an epidemic of obesity and diabetes, and frighteningly, there are now epidemic levels of childhood obesity. The link between obesity and diabetes is irrefutable. Since 1996 the number of people with diabetes in the UK has risen from 1.4 million to 2.9 million. Diabetes' prevalence in the UK is expected to rise to 4 million by 2025.

Insulin resistance is a precursor to diabetes, and may also lead to high cholesterol, high blood pressure and increased heart disease. Regardless of fertility, eating a correct diet for insulin balance is vital to your overall health, and insulin balance is VITAL to the balance of your fertility hormones.

The job of insulin is to convert carbohydrate into glucose (a form of sugar) which is then further converted to glycogen. Remember, glucose is not simply what we think of as refined sugar, it is a necessary building block for the fuel - glycogen - that gives us our energy.

This is why carbohydrates are an important part of our diet. It is not just grains and cereals that make up the carbohydrate family: all the root vegetables, many other vegetables, plus all the pulses and all the legumes (peas and beans) are strong and valuable sources of necessary carbohydrates.

When cells are insensitive to insulin this is called 'insulin resistance', meaning that the glucose is not being processed, so the blood sugar remains at high levels within the bloodstream, rather than being converted and stored as glycogen. The pancreas keeps on pumping out more insulin in order to try and control the levels of glucose in the bloodstream.

This leads to an excess of insulin in the bloodstream, and this is called *insulin resistance* because the body is resisting the insulin, ie. the insulin is not able to convert the glucose. High levels of insulin in the blood result when we eat highly refined carbohydrates, especially when we eat refined sugar.

Symptoms of insulin resistance may include:

- Fatigue and/or sleepiness
- Brain fogginess
- Low blood sugar (feeling agitated, jittery and/or moody with almost immediate relief once food is eaten)
- Constant hunger
- Cravings for sugars
- Falling asleep after meals
- Migrating aches and pains
- Intestinal bloating
- Increased weight and fat storage (despite dieting – the kind of weight that won't shift)
- Increased weight around the upper abdomen, often characterised by a heavy abdomen with slim hips and legs
- Increased triglycerides (the main constituent of body fat, measured by your doctor)
- Increased blood pressure
- Depression
- Skin tags
- Acanthosis nigricans (darkening of the skin especially in the neck and armpits).

If you think that you may have two or more of the symptoms of insulin resistance it is important to contact your GP and ask for a glucose-fasting test. This must be done by a medical professional and insulin resistance will be analysed by a blood test after a period of controlled fasting.

This blood test will measure your triglyceride and HDL (high-density lipoprotein) cholesterol levels, and will help to determine if you have a clinically significant level of insulin resistance. It is important to rule out if you may have Syndrome X, a metabolic condition (with a very strong genetic component) that can have a significant impact on ovulatory function. Many women with PCOS (polycystic ovarian syndrome) have insulin resistance. Insulin resistance will also affect spermatogenesis, so it is just as vital for men to get this tested.

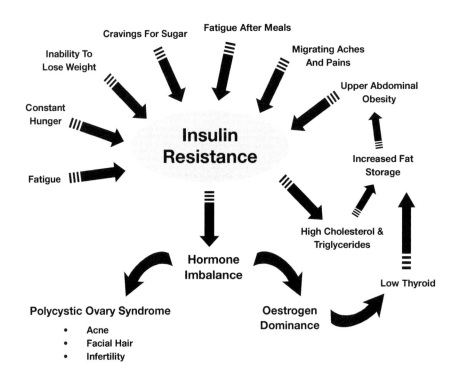

It is important to pay attention to this symptom list, for even if your blood tests come back in normal ranges, if you have these symptoms it may indicate that your body is struggling to metabolise your glucose levels properly.

Proper attention to a wholefood and a low GI diet is paramount to a healthy hormone balance. Give your digestion the workout it deserves and help to keep your digestion in great condition. If it isn't food as nature intended, then it probably isn't the right sort of food to be eating – this is a simple rule of thumb.

Luckily we are in the midst of 'clean food' revolution and now seeing a much improved culture of quality foods more available at the convenience level. So if you are eating on the run keep an eye out for (UK) chains such as Pret and Leon's. With the supermarket convenience foods please read the ingredients! If it has anything in it that isn't a real food, and it's not a wholefood with low GI, put it back on the shelf.

The best food discipline is to ensure that your kitchen cupboards and your fridge are only filled with nutritious vital foods that will enhance your libido and your fertility. Learning to eat in this way will bring you many health benefits, and it is a sure-fire preventative dietary approach that will keep you in good health your whole life long.

Be inspired! You are what you eat.

Your fertility – insulin imbalance and SHBG

High levels of insulin or spiking / crashing levels of blood sugar can really affect fertility, so we need to discuss SHBG (sex hormone-binding globulin) and the key reason why our insulin balance is vital to our fertility hormones.

SHBG is a protein molecule that acts as an escort for our sexual and reproductive hormones, ensuring that they do not exert their biological effects all of the time on all tissues. SHBG helps to carry your sex/conception hormones to exactly where they need to go, in the right levels, at the right frequency and in the right timing.

It is SHBG that helps to keep our HPO doing exactly what it should do, helping to keep us in regular healthy ovulation, and helping to ensure healthy sperm production.

When there is too much insulin in the bloodstream this will inhibit the production of SHBG. This is bad news for your fertility. Now SHBG is androgenic, meaning that it will pick up the androgen hormones, testosterone to be exact, before it will pick up the oestrogenic hormones, so lowered SHBG levels can have a significant effect on ovarian function which can lead to ovulation problems.

In men this will have a negative influence on sperm production (which relies on the LH and oestrogens as well as testosterone). Lowered SHBG also means that there will be lowered amount of testosterone reaching the gonads, thus libido will fall – always an issue when trying to deliver sperm!

Both men and women have *both* androgenic and oestrogenic hormones. Both men and women need to take care of their digestive balance in order to have a good fertility balance. The balance of these androgens and oestrogens are our hormones of sexuality, fired by our neurotransmitters of desire – dopamine and oxytocin – thus the balance of our libido depends on the balance of our digestion.

You are what you eat, and one of the sure-fire ways to improving your libido is to improve the balance of your blood sugar.

The Importance of BMI
– his and hers

Body Mass Index, BMI, is the ratio between your weight and your height, and used to determine if your weight is in a healthy range. Anything below 18.5 is too low, and anything above 25 is too high. Over 30 is considered obese, over 35 severely obese and over 40 is morbidly obese.

Being underweight is just as detrimental to your fertility as being overweight, and it is important to target any weight management to help you fall between 18.5–25.

BMI is calculated by dividing your height squared into your weight. There are many websites that can help you to do this calculation: try *www.nhs.uk/chq/Pages/how-can-i-work-out-my-bmi.aspx?CategoryID=51*.

If you are struggling to make this calculation then please make an appointment with the practice nurse at your GP surgery and they will be able to calculate your BMI.

Being overweight or underweight can affect your fertility and many of the studies done by many different IVF units clearly show a correlation between lower pregnancy rates in women with a BMI over 25, and that the miscarriage rates for women in this range are higher. Miscarriage is 4 times greater in women with a BMI over 30.

Being overweight can lead to complications for both mother and baby. Mothers are at increased risk of hypertension, a risk factor of pre-eclampsia, of gestational diabetes, of blood clots (DVT) and of Caesarean section as labours can be prolonged and more difficult.

There is also an increased risk for post-partum haemorrhage and infection and there is more chance of a urinary tract infection. UTI during gestation can be threatening for the baby.

Babies of overweight mothers have an increased risk of macrosomia, meaning they may be too large for a natural birth, which increases the chances of early induction and/or C-section delivery. These babies are at greater risk of neural tube defects (such as spina bifida) and more prone to suffer childhood obesity.

Underweight women will very often have sporadic ovulation and may move further towards anovulation (no ovulation) the more weight they lose. This is part of our bodies' inbuilt physiologic survival mechanism, as we need enough weight to bear a healthy pregnancy; our reserves of fat and protein molecules are vital, particularly in the first trimester when the body is constructing the placenta.

Underweight pregnancies have a higher risk of premature delivery, and there is a higher risk of having a 'small for dates baby' meaning that the baby may be malnourished for their particular developmental stage, which may lead to health complications as they grow and mature.

It is so important to understand these implications.

This is about so much more than just being able to get pregnant, it is also about the health of your pregnancy and the health of your baby. Paying attention to your BMI is a vital aspect of your journey to conceive, and I urge you to look carefully at your weight and your partner's.

The symptom lists for insulin resistance, for stress responses and for low thyroid can be quite interchangeable, and all of these things affect our fertility hormone balance. If you are experiencing any of the symptoms already listed, please see your GP and discuss if you should have the blood tests that will assess your metabolic markers.

It is really worth your while to make sure that your metabolism is in good condition, and to pay careful attention to eating a balancing diet. It is worth your time and money to invest in a good nutritionist so as to take care of your digestive metabolism. This will serve you in all aspects of your well-being, for your libido and help to protect your future health.

You are what you eat, and your gametes are what you eat, and those gametes are that embryo, that foetus, that baby, that infant, that child, that teenager ...

How you eat *now* is an investment, not only in your own future health but also in the health of your baby.

Right, enough evangelism for one chapter! Let's take a look at just two of the digestive metabolic markers (there are hundreds). This is to give you a mere glimpse at the elegantly poetic way the body's endocrine system (the body's collection of glands that produce hormones with a number of functions) and neurotransmission (that is, the transmission of our nerve impulses) are constantly orchestrating the most complex symphony imaginable.

Your endocrine is managed through a finely balanced system of feedback loops that consistently trigger your hormonal messaging into a sequence that keeps you in balance.

This exquisite symphony is your metabolism.

Losing weight safely to keep digestive balance

For all the reasons we have discussed in the previous chapters, our digestive balance is paramount to the healthy balance of our fertility hormones. When we have a weight imbalance, this can have detrimental effects on our leptin, a hormone, and on our adiponectin, a protein, both of which are vital to our digestive structure and metabolism.

I don't wish to blind you with the biochemistry, so in a nutshell I can tell you that when our leptin and adiponectin are out of balance this will disrupt our fertility hormones. Crash dieting creates a yo-yo effect as it plays havoc with our leptin feedback loops, for as the leptin levels drop this tells the body to conserve its fat tissues.

This is why crash diets will *never* work and they are also very detrimental to your fertility. Trying to control our weight by restricting our calorific intake will cause the leptin levels to fall, increasing our stress response and lowering or even switching off our HPO feedback loops.

When we carry too much weight our adiponectin levels will also drop, and this can affect our insulin sensitivity. People with lowered adiponectin will be more prone to insulin resistance, and thus have less SHBG, and so the fine-tuned balance that our HPO relies on will be disrupted.

So in summary, insulin resistance will affect the leptin and adiponectin levels, and changes in the leptin and adiponectin will affect the insulin resistance. It can be a bit chicken and egg, for insulin resistance will lead to carrying excess abdominal weight, which can lead to crash dieting, and then leads to disrupted leptins (as does being underweight). This eventually leads to dropped adiponectin levels, as the body conserves its fat reserves, and leads back to insulin resistance.

It is just as important for healthy sperms that men also have a well-managed weight within the normal BMI range. If you are carrying a bit of extra poundage coupled with poor sperm parameters then have your metabolism tested to check that your insulin is in balance. Your blood test results may come back in the normal range (please pay attention if they are near the borders of the normal range), but if you are having insulin resistance symptoms your normal fertility function may be disrupted. If you have any of the symptoms listed earlier, please consider an insulin-balancing low GI wholefood approach to eating.

To reiterate, for both men and women, digestive balance is vital to fertility.

If you are carrying too much weight I suggest you seek professional advice from a good nutritionist who is a specialist in fertility, and can help you to structure a low-GI insulin-balancing approach to taking the weight off. The safest rate to reduce weight is at 1 pound per week (sorry, old money, err ... 2.2 kilos).

Remember that crash diets only seem to work because they mostly just shed the fluid retention that many overweight people have, but there is no foundation in these diets and they will play havoc with your metabolic balance.

This isn't about suggesting a diet that is about losing weight. What I am suggesting is that you permanently change your eating habits. Your body will naturally begin to better metabolise and the weight will go.

I have had insulin resistance since my teens, coupled with a thyroid imbalance, PCOS and endometriosis. When it comes to understanding hormone imbalances I have very first-hand experience! I began to change my diet as a result of studying the metabolism of digestion and fertility, and as my metabolism improved, the weight just melted away. I lost 4 dress sizes without even trying. Though I wasn't trying to get pregnant, for the first time in four decades I had a balanced metabolism, no more hormonal mood swings, bundles of vitality, and a, ahem, very healthy libido!

Low blood sugar – hypoglycaemia

When the blood sugar is too low then we may feel symptoms indicating that the glucose levels in the bloodstream are too low to properly fuel us.

Low blood sugar is called hypoglycaemia and can give us symptoms such as:

- Headache
- Hunger
- Nervousness
- Drowsiness
- Dizziness
- Irritability
- Shaking
- Sweating
- Weakness
- Palpitations.

High blood sugar – hyperglycaemia

Classic symptoms:

- Frequently hungry (polyphagia)
- Frequently thirsty (polydipsia)
- Frequently urinating (polyuria)

Other symptoms:

- Blurred vision
- Fatigue
- Weight loss
- Poor wound healing (cuts, scrapes, etc.)
- Dry mouth
- Dry or itchy skin
- Impotence
- Recurrent infections (such as vaginal thrush, groin rash, external ear infection).

Diabetes

Type 2 Diabetes Mellitis (T2DM): the body is insensitive to normal amounts of insulin, leading to an excess in the bloodstream, and is not able to control blood sugar levels.

Type 1 Diabetes Mellitis (T1DM): the body is not producing enough insulin to control blood sugar levels.

Either way, there is too much glucose in the bloodstream.

It is important to remember that the symptoms of insulin disorders, stress responses and thyroid disorder are all quite similar, and in many cases inter-related. Insulin resistance is not necessarily connected to your weight, as weight loss and the inability to put weight on may be due to other metabolic disorders.

As you read through all this endocrine discussion, if you feel that you have some of these symptoms (for stress, insulin resistance, thyroid), please see your GP to discuss if you should have some metabolic testing.

Thyroid balance is vital *for your fertility*

The thyroid is one of the most important endocrine glands in the body, and it exerts its hormonal influence on every aspect of our physiology: our digestion, our nervous system, our circulatory system and of course, our sexual/reproductive system.

Thyroid hormones affect every cell in the body, and their primary purpose is to encourage protein production, as well as stimulating the energy-producing cells that energise our bodies.

Having an underactive thyroid (hypothyroid) can inhibit ovulation. Decreased thyroxine (a vital hormone for our reproductive function) can also affect the progesterone levels, which can lead to a shortened luteal phase, which in turn inhibits implantation.

In men a hypothyroid will affect libido, as the volume of sex hormones will decrease, meaning that sperm and testosterone production will fall. Men with low thyroid parameters tend to have low libido and low sperm parameters.

With an overactive thyroid (hyperthyroid) the body is doing the opposite, sending the body into a state of over-activity. This can have a detrimental effect on ovulation, causing irregular cycles or even anovulation.

The treatment of hyperthyroid during pregnancy must be managed with care by a specialist endocrinologist who is an expert in thyroid treatment, as there are risks to the baby's thyroid development, and there are increased risks of miscarriage, premature birth and low birth weight.

If you are concerned that you may have symptoms of thyroid imbalance, keep in mind that many cross over with the stress and insulin resistance symptoms. Please see your GP or your fertility consultant.

I have been treating fertility for 17 years now, and it is completely fair to say that these simple metabolic markers may often be overlooked or not investigated until there have been recurrent miscarriages or repeated failed IVFs. These other metabolic markers (thyroid, stress hormones) are seldom investigated when there is a diagnosis of unexplained infertility. Our endocrine balance, our digestive balance and our emotional balance are the 3 primary foundations for all the systems that govern conception. Endocrine function *IS* the Fizz.

Symptoms of hypothyroid (underactive)

- Tiredness
- Weight gain
- Feeling cold
- Dry skin
- Lifeless hair
- Fluid retention
- Mental sluggishness
- Depression
- Hoarse voice
- Irregular menstruation

- Heavy periods
- Low libido
- Infertility
- Carpal tunnel syndrome
- Memory loss.

Symptoms of hyperthyroid (overactive)

- Feeling nervous, restless, emotional, irritable
- Raised blood pressure
- Sleeping poorly
- Hand tremor
- Losing weight despite increased appetite
- Palpitations
- Sweating
- Disliking heat
- Increased thirst
- Diarrhoea
- Frequent urgency to move bowels
- Shortness of breath
- Itchy skin
- Thinning hair
- Light or infrequent periods
- Tiredness
- Muscle weakness
- Goitre (swelling of the thyroid)
- Swelling of the eyes (exophthalmos – see Marty Feldman).

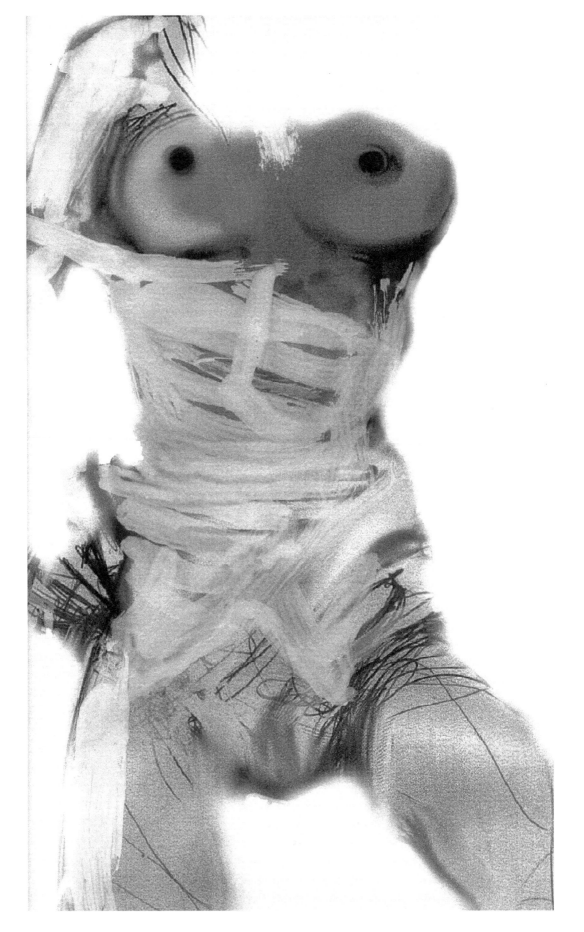

moonwashed

the full moon light casts iridescent blue white
i stand beneath and feel magnetic pull
my cells and fluids course and reach
drawn by the magic that sources my centre

moonlight
moonpath
moonsong
i am of your night
mostly deeply my true self
when bathed in the wash of your currents

and the exquisite thrill
of this liaison
this moonwashed attraction
rises in me like a tide
and i must away to my chamber
to lie upon my bed and dream of this lover
this libertine who has swept into my life
opening a chamber within me
to the hidden delights and darkest fruits
of my deepest longings

this lover who will share without boundaries
unfettered fettered wild exploration
of a like-spirit
kindred in the need for this touch
to be touched
he who has known me
who knows my soft fingers

so wanting
to caress with delight the length of that blade
i am awash in the need to feel that hardened shaft
pulsing and flicking with anticipation

as you lie upon the bed, i straddle over you
the silkiness of my thighs perched gently on yours
skin pricks electric
my arms stretch forward
holding your wrists pinioned

slowly i dip
the exquisite softness of my breasts
nestle against your inner thigh
my hair gently sways upon your skin
and like a leaf from a tree
i drop
into the soft fold
into the hollow of your groin
to breathe in the potent scent of you
your musk radiating
drawing me to take you

my gentle breath blows hot into your hollow
searing through your skin into the deep core
pulling, magnetic
your hardened shaft
swells harder
and the length of you is sentinel
as the tip of my tongue
dips to your skin
swirling

and your indrawn breath lances through me
like fire in my veins

i am charged with the need to feel you
and my head swirls towards you
finding the rooted fold
nuzzling the softness of my cheek on the silky taut skin of you
and with deliberate slowness
tantalise upward
soft brushes, merest whisper of touch
finding your contours
your pathways and tributaries
the map of you

i feel your thighs tightening
your stillness so erotic
as we plunder with merest movement
into sensations of feeling
each other's self

i rise and rise, so gently, so slowly
ever reaching for the glorious crest
finding that ridge
learning the swoop of your camber
the convex and concave of you
and still my lips have not touched you
and the aching want of the need
seeps a pearl of moisture

and i lift my head
now above you
your glistening blade proud and full

as i fall
straight down upon the tip of you to lick the fluid of your wanting

and in a cascade my lips slide down on every side of you
slipping my mouth around you, gathering the rim of your helmet within my
embracing lips
and then
soft tug as i slowly pull upward
the suctioned draw pulling deep
swelling your already engorged member
to a judder of bursting need

and the fury is upon me

to feel every millimetre of your shaft
lips and tongue, tracing, racing
upwards and down
all the while your helmet strains
desperate to feel again those encompassing lips descend upon you

your wrists lift, straining against the weight of my bearing arms
i plunge down upon you, deep and full, you are swallowed in my delight
and i stroke up and down
long deep swallows
feeling your bursting fullness

suddenly
in the drive of overwhelming need
you lift and flip me and i am impaled by the sheathing of your blade
sudden and swift you enter me
with your own fury to explode
surging slicing strokes

ramming to the hilt
driving driving drilling upward
stroke swift stroke
plunging, like diving into the embracing sea
cascading into shuddering release

i feel the hot pump of your seed as it hits the roof of me
wave after wave
as my very self grips to every part of you
feeling the fluids within you surge and surge upward to spill within me

aftershocks
causing me to quiver and jolt
and i spasm around your member
panting, delighted
slowly returning
catching breath as heartbeats gentle and the languid draws our limbs into
heaviness

and as you slip out of me
in a burst of further delight
i whirl round
reach down

and lick you clean

and like the cat that caught the canary
i grin

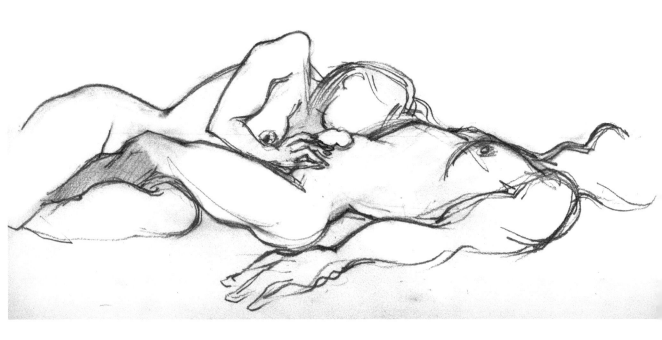

Chapter Eighteen

Caffeine – our barista whizzy culture

Bang one up baby (an automatic double shot, that is). Every barista coffee *is* going to be a double shot, that's standard.

We live in a culture that is very caffeine driven. Tea, coffee, hot chocolate, sodas, and now these 'energising' drinks. Many over-the-counter cold and flu pharmaceutical remedies include caffeine, as do many of the analgesics (headache tablets). Everywhere we look we are being offered these stimulants to help us cruise through our daily grind. Except they are very detrimental to our overall health, and give a false boost of energy that actually, in the long run, drains us of our fundamental well-being and genuine energy.

How did we become such a coffee culture? Isn't it interesting to note that the rise of the coffee culture matches the dawning and subsequent blanketing of the Internet culture? Our modern world is fast, and caffeine is a very speedy stimulant. It seems that it helps us keep up with the pace we have generated.

So how does caffeine affect our fertility? There is a spectrum of information about how it affects our physiology, but for our purposes let us focus on the way that caffeine imposes on both our sympathetic response, and ways it specifically affects our reproduction.

There is an overall recognition that taking caffeine is detrimental to fertility, though constant studies have not yet revealed a single firm conclusion. Some studies show that moderate caffeine (less than 300 mg day, or about 3 cups of coffee) does not adversely affect ovulation. Other studies show that moderate caffeine intake slightly delays the onset of pregnancy and poses a small risk to the developing child. Caffeine enters the fallopian tubes and uterus, as it does most every other tissue in the body. Caffeine has been found in newly fertilised embryos. Caffeine crosses the placenta, showing an increase in the baby's heart rate and changes in the foetal movement patterns.

The Nurses' Health Study done in America in 1989 showed that women who had more than 400 mg caffeine daily were 20 per cent more likely to experience trouble conceiving.

This may be due to the caffeine making the fallopian tubes less able to relax and contract, thus slowing the passage of the embryo in reaching the endometrium. There are studies to show that caffeine makes the endometrium less hospitable and that a lot of caffeine every day *may* increase the risks of miscarriage, premature delivery and low birth weight, although there is no rock-solid proof of this.

Caffeine also affects our adrenals and impacts our autonomic systems, affecting our sympathetic response – with a corresponding knock-on effect on both our digestive and reproductive feedback loops (bang-bang-bang sound her drums).

Add a dose or two of sugar to your coffee, and then we also need to think about the way this can affect our blood sugar balance – particularly on an empty stomach first thing in the morning (what?! Start the day without a cup of coffee/tea!?) as many of us do.

Caffeine is considered to be a psychoactive substance, meaning that it crosses the blood-brain barrier and acts on the central nervous system, generating a change in mood. In the case of coffee, it often brings an increased sense of alertness and endurance.

Caffeine is classed as a stimulant, along with amphetamine, cocaine and nicotine. Caffeine is actually classified as a drug. Its side effects include headache, insomnia, restlessness, agitation and tremors. It stimulates adrenalin, which is both a hormone and neurotransmitter, affecting the heart and liver cells, increasing heart rate and stimulating the conversion of glycogen to glucose (thus raising the blood sugar levels).

Caffeine interferes with a neurotransmitter called adenosine (which suppresses neural activity in the brain), whose job it is to let us know when we feel tired. Adenosine increases blood flow throughout the body and is an important part of our metabolic balance.

So contrary to popular belief, caffeine does not give you more energy, and it does not speed up your metabolism. It can block your body's self-regulation, and in long-term overuse of caffeine suppresses your metabolism and can lead to adrenal fatigue.

The jury is absolutely out in respect of whether caffeine inhibits fertility, but these studies are usually done in the context of the direct effect on the ovulation, fallopian patency (how well the sperms and embryo can travel within the tubes), and on the effect it may have in the endometrium.

Without question caffeine does disrupt your metabolic balance, this evidence is crystal clear. As we begin to recognise that we get pregnant with our whole body, we also need to respect that caffeine does have a significant impact and can affect our hormonal feedback loops.

So how much caffeine is OK?

I always ask people to come off a coffee habit nice and slowly. For people who have a regular use of 400+ mg per day (or around 4 cups a day), they are likely to experience the following:

Coffee withdrawal symptoms

- Chills and/or hot spells
- Decreased alertness
- Depressed mood
- Difficulty concentrating or thinking
- Digestive issues (usually constipation, but sometimes also nausea and / or vomiting)
- Fatigue, lethargy and / or sleepiness
- Headaches, ranging from moderate to severe, and usually starting behind the eyes before spreading
- Irritability (moderate to extreme) and restlessness
- Insomnia (although it seems counter-intuitive, this can be an issue for some people!)
- Muscle stiffness and / or pain
- Sinus issues (usually blocked sinuses or cold-like symptoms).

(See *http://coffeetea.about.com/od/caffeinehealth/a/Caffeine-Withdrawal-Symptoms.htm*)

Most of the fertility websites suggest that the appropriate amount of caffeine when you are trying to conceive is less than 200 mg per day (or 2 cups).

If you are struggling to give up that one important cup of tea or coffee, please drink it after you have eaten, so that your blood sugar is more stable before you take the caffeine that will stimulate the glycogen conversion. The more stable your blood sugar, the better your reproductive feedback loops will behave.

I believe it is just as important to pay attention to quality. Organic coffee is much less toxic, and Fair-trade products help the economy of the coffee growers, so this brings very good energy to your purchasing power and enhances the value of the coffee you are drinking.

Decaffeinated coffee has a significantly reduced caffeine, with about 97 per cent removed. The recommended process is the 'Swiss water method' as this has the best flavour retention. The chemical process of removing the caffeine was toxic once upon a time but these methods have long been dropped and now decaffeinating methods are relatively benign. Quality is the message, so water-stripped organic decaf is the best.

In my opinion, instant coffee is generally *toxic*. Full stop. Please do not drink this product, as the chemicals used to render the coffee into the freeze-dried state are detrimental to your health on every level.

The caffeine milligram content in tea, coffee, chocolate and sodas

Coffee:

- Filtered (8 oz) = 234 mg
- Percolated (8 oz) = 176 mg
- Instant (8 oz) = 85 mg
- Decaffeinated instant (8 oz) = 3 mg
- Expresso (1–2 oz) = 45-100 mg
- Starbucks grande (16 oz) = 330 mg

Tea:

- One-minute brew = 9–33 mg
- Three-minute brew = 20–46 mg
- Canned iced tea (12 oz) = 22–36 mg

Soft drinks:

- Dr Pepper = 39.6 mg
- Cola = 46 mg
- Diet cola = 46 mg

Cocoa and chocolate:

- Cocoa (6 oz) = 10 mg
- Milk chocolate (1 oz) = 6 mg
- Baking chocolate (1 oz) = 35 mg

See *http://infertility.about.com/od/researchandstudies/a/caffeine_fertility.htm*

Alcohol – how much is too much?

You will recall that my colleague Mr Dooley rang me concerned that I seemed to be counselling couples that it was OK to have a drink, when the received wisdom is that if you are trying to conceive then alcohol is best avoided.

I absolutely concur with this advice. Drinking is rarely beneficial for our health, and drinking excessively is very definitely detrimental for our health. Equally, moderate imbibing will cause no discernible harm. So I believe that occasionally getting a bit tiddly (but never drunk) on champagne benefits our hearts and minds, for it is good to look forward to a lovely treat at a time when we may be feeling at our most keyed-up and tense.

Ovum

So what do the studies say about the effects of alcohol on female fertility?

I'm afraid we are back to that proverbial piece of string, for you will find many conflicting bits of 'evidence'. Although there is no conclusive evidence that taking an occasional drink will inhibit fertility, an article recently published in the British Medical Journal suggested that women who drink socially 1–5 units per week showed reduced fertility compared to women who drank nothing at all.

According to the Nurses' Health Study, problems with ovulation were no more common in the group of women who had a moderate intake of one drink per day than those who didn't drink.

Given this uncertainty around alcohol and reproduction, the safest course of action is to forgo alcohol when trying to conceive.

I particularly suggest this advice with my Chinese medicine hat on. Each of us has a unique constitutional diagnosis, and each of us has weak links within our physiology. Some of us will metabolise alcohol easily enough and it will not put much of a strain upon our systems. Others will be more susceptible to alcohol, and it will undermine and inhibit our optimum function, and for some of us just one drink can place too much strain on our liver function which ultimately will be detrimental to our fertility.

This is a key factor in Chinese diagnostics, as the Liver channel system governs the menstruation and the smooth flow of the blood and Qi. Any woman who is suffering menstrual discomforts or irregularities should be aware that alcohol will potentially have a negative effect.

So you must never take alcohol when you are pregnant, ergo, you should never take alcohol during your luteal phase (which is between the time when you ovulate, and when you get your period). Your sperms and ovum are that baby, so avoiding alcohol will contribute to the health of your embryo.

Sperms

So we have heard that very moderate drinking does not seem to affect ovulation, but what about those sperms?

Without doubt any amount of drinking is detrimental to sperm development, and binge drinking is the worst possible scenario and kills them off in droves.

In this the evidence is very clear, for it is easy to measure. Repeat sperm analysis shows that alcohol will *always* have a detrimental effect on sperm development, and it will affect both the sperm count (concentration) and quality (the morphology, or shapes), which will affect how they move (motility).

Alcohol metabolism will use up the body's reserves of zinc, and zinc is one of the key minerals in the development of sperm. Please don't kid yourself into thinking that you can just take a zinc supplement and drink as much as you like; our body's ability to absorb and balance nutrients is a very complex process that relies on a fine balance of all the right ingredients in all the right proportions to each other in order to properly metabolise.

If you are stepping out of a drinking lifestyle in order to try and conceive, it is super important to pay attention to your nutritional balance. Wherever possible please find a well qualified nutritionist to help you analyse your nutritional status and to ensure that you are taking the correct kinds of supplements.

If cost is an issue, find a good antenatal broad-spectrum supplement, and for men look for the many male fertility complexes that are now available. See the Useful Resources section for some recommendations.

Every kind of alcohol is very high in sugar, but beer and wine are most especially high, and we now know how detrimental it is to our insulin balance to flood the systems with sugar spikes. High levels of insulin will affect the SHBG, which will affect the HPG (hypothalamus-pituitary-gonadal axis) which *will affect* sperm development – whether this is regular or binge drinking.

Regarding my advice for the tiddly bonk at ovulation, I am absolutely not advocating that either of you should get drunk. The amount of alcohol shared at this time should have such a minimal impact as to be negligible.

Chinese medicine again: as it is for women, the Liver channel system is an important player in the fertility of men, and there is no question that alcohol taxes the body at the level of the liver. If the liver organ is trying to metabolise alcohol, this will compromise its function in the governance of the development of healthy sperm.

The same advice applies for men as women as regards our capacity to metabolise alcohol. For many people, our drinking culture is just a normal way of life, and the signs and symptoms of a hangover are normal, and many of us have become quite adept at ignoring that the alcohol we drink is impacting negatively on our ability to function.

Remember please that if a hangover is making you feel so bad that you are needing to take an analgesic (painkiller) or it is making you shake, feel nauseous or impairing your balance or judgement, these are clear signs that you have crossed over your body's line in its ability to appropriately metabolise the alcohol.

If you are drinking to the extent of vomiting, this should be regarded as alcohol-poisoning, as your body is working to eject the toxin that it does not have the power to fully metabolise.

Many of the signs and symptoms of a hangover are much more subtle, and I ask you to really pay attention to how you feel the morning after having a few drinks as opposed to the morning after no alcohol at all.

The symptoms of a hangover

According to the National Institute on Alcohol Abuse and Alcoholism, a hangover can include the following symptoms:

- Fatigue, weakness and thirst
- Headache and muscle aches
- Nausea, vomiting and stomach pain
- Decreased sleep
- Vertigo and sensitivity to light and sound
- Decreased attention and concentration
- Depression, anxiety and irritability
- Tremor, sweating, night sweats, and increased pulse and systolic blood pressure.

If you are suffering from any difficulty getting or holding an erection when under the influence of alcohol then it must be strenuously avoided. This is a case of paying attention to your physiology which is telling you that the alcohol is affecting your central nervous system. It goes without saying that no hard on = no ejaculation = no sperm = no conception.

To summarise, alcohol will never promote fertility. Please avoid alcohol altogether, but if it feels appropriate for you by all means chill that bottle of champers and at ovulation have a gently tiddly, celebratory take-a-break-from-being-perfect-all-of-the-time-take-the-edge-off kind of lovemaking that puts the emphasis back into being relaxed, care-free and loving for it's own sake.

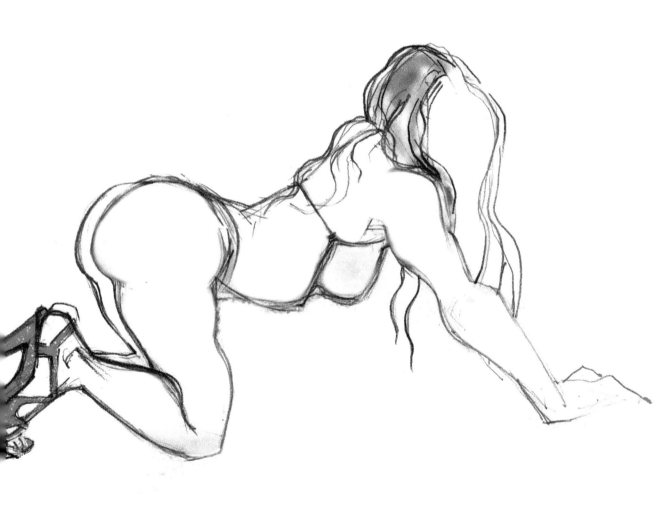

will you bite me?

with my peachy ass raised and quivering
will you bite me till i squeal?

shall i sit upon the bed in stockings and hooker heels
basque thrust breasts pushed high
raspberry nipples peaked and peeking
knees raised
my flower spread wide
as you watch me touch myself
my pink gash open to your gaze
my sensual fingering
inviting you to devour me?

will it make you want to ram me
hard against the wall
knifing your fingers into me
so the edge of subjugation makes me throw my head back in the delight of
your force?

will you spread my legs wide and lick my cunt until i am streaming with
juices so ripe and flowing
you cannot but sink your hand into me
straining my edges until i whimper?

will you like to hear me whimper?
to beg you to do those naughty things
to bind me to your will?

will you spank me as i bend over
my suspendered ass pulled taut by my leaning
begging for your touch
however you choose
me not knowing
quite what you will do?

will you look down upon my lowered head
your fingers tangled in my hair
and relish the way
i devour your cock?

will you drill me with your wanting
taking me hard and fast
rough and ready
harlot abandoned?

will you push me so hard that the edges of my fear make my eyes go wide?
not in fear of you
oh no lover libertine
i am not afraid of you

take me to the edges of my boundaries and push me

if i need you to pull me back i know that you will

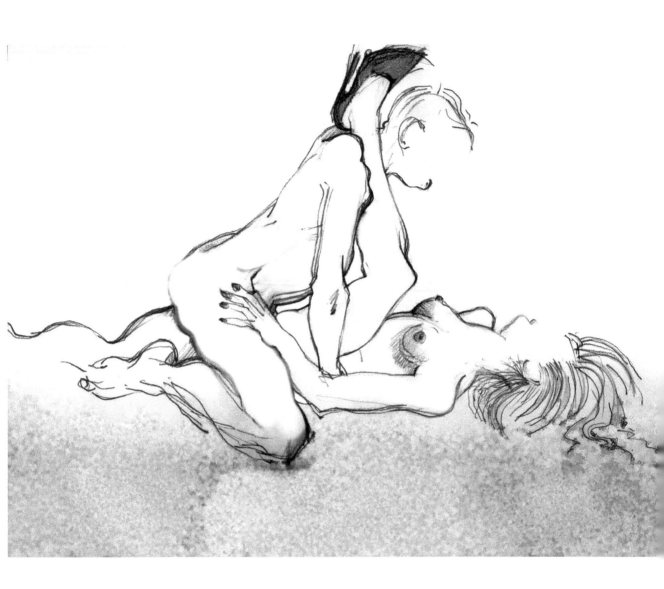

Chapter Nineteen

Getting pregnant – yikes! The first trimester – love and fear – again!

There is this amazing contradiction in seeing that positive test, for just as we have achieved the longed-for result and the joy and excitement courses through us, almost instantaneously we feel doubt and fear as we think, 'oh my, please, please, please let this be a healthy pregnancy!'

Yet again we find ourselves caught in the loop of the cycle of hope and fear, the switchy thing is fully at play, and we can easily teeter-totter between our sympathetic and parasympathetic. It is so important for us to remain in our parasympathetic, and yet the fears that accompany the first trimester are likely to push us into that sympathetic response.

Let me reassure you that the fears women experience in the first trimester are normal, and every woman has them, regardless of her conception circumstances. But when it has taken many months/years to conceive, when this is an IVF conception, if we have had a previous miscarriage ... all of this can heighten and emphasise those normal fears into a much higher resonance.

The best advice I can offer is to recognise that the most important thing to do is:

just be pregnant until there is any evidence otherwise.

Easier said than done, *but* I can assure you that how we think and feel in these early weeks is an important part of helping this to become a nurturing pregnancy.

If we spend all our time on tenterhooks, startling with every twinge, constantly imagining that every little thing we may be feeling might be something wrong, then we are sure to be pushing ourselves into that state of chronic sympathetic.

Your body is building a placenta! Think of your lower pelvis as being like a massive construction site, say, a whole city block turning into an underground car park and shopping centre with a huge set of tower blocks above with a landscaped street concourse.

Think about the finely tuned orchestration of how services and construction supplies need to be sequenced in order for all of the infrastructure to be in place before the buildings start to appear. Think of the site management that is required as delivery after delivery brings in the materials that will step by step contribute to the overall construction.

All of the twinges and pulls and tugs, the sensations we can feel in those first tenterhook weeks, these are the normal sensations that reflect the astonishing amount of site management that is going on as your body builds the equivalent of that city block complex. And there is no way to differentiate the way that these sensations feel from the way our menstrual symptoms feel. It is the same, because it is all the same organs and membranes, muscles and ligaments that are involved in this new process.

It is so easy to allow the fears and doubts to have the upper hand, and to hold ourselves back from the joy and delight just in case it doesn't work. It's just the same as the mechanism we might use when we are trying to conceive, believing that if we hold back then somehow it will not be as disappointing *if it doesn't work*.

We discussed this in detail in earlier, and I promise you, any miscarriage will bring The Disappointment, and no amount of holding yourself back from the *joy* of being pregnant will actually change the devastation if the pregnancy does not progress.

Allowing yourself to flow in the Joy, the Delight, the Wonder, allowing your-self to feel the Thrill, the Excitement, the Marvellous Sense of Accomplish-ment – these are the feelings that welcome this pregnancy. *Pregnancy is a receptive process*. If we allow ourselves to be fully receptive we will embrace all the potential of this pregnancy.

Miscarriage is a *normal* part of pregnancy. We have also covered this, and I encourage you to recognise and embrace that you must gracefully concede to nature's wisdom, and while you are waiting to see if this is indeed a viable pregnancy, then opening your heart and receiving and welcoming the poten-tial of the person who may be entering your lives is a vital and important part of being pregnant.

Time and time again I have held hands with women who are desperately hold-ing themselves back from connecting to the pregnancy just in case it will not work. Although it feels immensely counter-intuitive, I assure you that if you open your heart and embrace the pregnancy, if it does need to be a miscarriage then your openness will give you the resilience to better cope with the loss.

Reduced anxiety happens when we are in parasympathetic, and when we are in parasympathetic then our oxytocin can flow.

What oxytocin does for the body:

- Increase calmness and has a sleep-inducing effect
- Reduce pain
- Enhance social memory (or shared social histories)
- Help the person becomes more nurturing
- Enhance bonding
- Improve the ability to learn and increases curiosity
- Reduce blood pressure
- Balance body temperature
- Regulate digestion
- Regulate fluid levels
- Increase the body's ability to heal and grow
- Reduce muscle tension

and most importantly,

- Reduce anxiety.

So the answer to the first trimester of walking on those eggshells of apprehension and fear is to do whatever you can to nurture your oxytocin, to feel grounded in the *belonging* that we have with our lover, as we bravely step into the unknown in sure heart that if this is the child that is meant to be, all will be well.

Remember, just be pregnant until there is any evidence otherwise ...

Revel in the delight of your conception. I won't say drink champagne – but metaphorically speaking, let yourselves flow in the river of the golden bubbles of celebration. Be Thrilled. Be Excited. Be Ecstatically Happy.

Let those hormones of your happiness Fizz up the conception to the fullness of its capacity.

It is certainly a time of deep excitement, sometimes so deep that we hardly dare let ourselves feel it. So take a deep breath, release your solar plexus, let the joy in your heart flow to the uterus, and just be. Just be pregnant.

I am compelled to repeat: you really cannot analyse those tweaks and twinges. All the muscles, ligaments, vessels, membranes and organs that are involved in sexuality, menstruation, reproduction, are exactly the same muscles, ligaments, vessels and organs that are now the construction site of this pregnancy, and are the exact same muscles that will help you birth this child. You genuinely cannot differentiate what may be a construction twinge from what might be a potential miscarriage.

Those site managers have a lot of sequencing and sorting to do!

The Importance of Reassurance

I spend a lot of time with TTC women in their first trimester, and have some sense of the accompanying anxieties that come with the minefield of trying to get pregnant, especially the arduous against-the-odds IVF kind of conception.

I always encourage these women to come in regularly through the first trimester (thinking back to that St Mary's study I mentioned in the introduction) for the incredible value that reassuring support can bring.

There was a study done at St Mary's Hospital London in 1989, and the results were so surprising they repeated the study again just to be sure. This was a recurrent miscarriage study.

The control group were given standard care, which consists of a scan between 6–8 weeks, followed by a scan again at 12 weeks. The study group was offered reassurance care, which consisted of coming in to the hospital once a week, up until 12 weeks, to spend half an hour in a room with a person, talking about their thoughts and feelings, their fears and concerns. There was no touching, no physical intervention at all. The only treatment was a listening ear.

At the end of 12 weeks the 'standard care' control group had a pregnancy rate of 29%, which is about normal for the parameters of the expected conception rates, as between 20–25% of embryos will implant to become a viable pregnancy.

The 'reassurance care' study group had a pregnancy rate of 87%. This result was so astonishing that the study was actually repeated, just to ensure that they were not looking at fluky results. When the study was repeated the results were virtually identical.

I have long been delighted by these studies, as they exemplify to me the very core of what can happen when we allow ourselves to accept and embrace our fears. When this happens our switches allow us to better remain in parasympathetic, and this is the resilience that gives us the capacity to cope with whatever will come what may.

Reassurance about diet in the first trimester

Every day seems to bring something new. You are still yourself, yet there is this chemical cocktail brewing that is making you feel more different than you have ever felt.

The way we experience a pregnancy depends on our pre-existing condition before the pregnancy, and will very much depend on how our systems are functioning and how they adapt to the onslaught of hormonal engineering that is building that 'whole city block' within us.

All of your preconception care is an *investment* in the health of your pregnancy. Every bit of being-ever-so-good will pay off in spades, and potentially lead to a relatively comfortable first trimester.

What is normal in the first trimester is *tiredness* (so get horizontal as often as you can – the blood returns to the organs and aids in the placental construction) and usually, though not always, there will be nausea. And with IVF it is common that the pregnancy will start with a lot of extra fluid and inflammation in the pelvic cavity from the stimulation treatment, so there may be excess bloating to contend with.

There are many symptoms we might talk about. Obstetric care is a whole book in itself (the next book in this series: *Birth-fit Fizz*), so I mustn't slide into that discussion here (this is really hard for me!). However, I do wish to suggest one significant titbit of advice that may set your mind at ease.

Many women are very concerned about their nutritional input in the first trimester, and when nausea and vomiting, appetite changes, food aversions, constipation and carb and sugar cravings begin to rule – they begin to feel a bit freaked out that all they can manage is white bread and butter.

Many women feel that they should be eating whole wheat, loads of green veg, all their low GI goodies, everything they know to be the right kinds of healthy foods.

Well actually, when the hormonal soup is playing havoc with your body chemistry and you find that only certain foods are all that you can manage, please trust that *this is just fine.*

What?! A whole berloody book that harps on about correct and vital nutrition – and now you are saying no worries, just eat what you can???

Yup.

Counter-intuitive queen, that's me.

In the first trimester, the time between 6–8 weeks when the placenta and the embryo plumb together is the biologically correct time for pregnancy nausea to arise. This is when there begins to be a flow from the placenta to the embryo, and a new and different directional flow within the maternal body. In Chinese medicine we call this *counterflow Qi.*

In addition to all that your body is doing to manage its own physiology, you now have a whole new super-highway's worth of extra function going on, all pouring in the direction of the uterus. That is usually at the root of the nausea: the swim of all those busy-busy hormones, and the building of that construction site.

In the context of this marvellous strangeness of feeling so different, the most important thing you can do is to take the path of least resistance and float through all the changes with as light an approach as you can, meaning the least exertion possible. Commuting and working will probably be all that you will want to manage, and sleep as much as you can, be horizontal whenever possible, and eat in a way that works for you.

My reassurance is simple. All the nutrition that you and your embryo/foetus need is amply stored within you, and your body will draw on its reserves of nutrition to sustain you through these chemical soup days.

This is one of the key reasons for the core advice throughout this book: to pay very close attention to your preconception nutritional input. You need to lay down the value in your stored nutritional reserves that will help to sustain you through these first 12 weeks.

What is important is to pay attention and respect your aversions and cravings. Absolutely 100 per cent avoid anything with additives and preservatives, this is *not* permission to eat *any* junk food, and watch out for those commercial breads and baked goods that are chock-full of stabilisers and preservatives, trans fats and refined sugars. You need quality, not crap.

What is important to respect is that you will need an astonishing amount of carbohydrates, and that often the more refined carbs are much better for you.

You need fast fuel that is very easy to digest. (Brown rice and lentils with greens at this stage of mega development are not going to be easy to digest!)

And you need to eat little and often. Uncomplicated food is the answer, in small portions. White bread and butter (toast!) is an ideal delivery of the fast carbs and saturated fat that you most need.

If you do have a healthy appetite for any of your normal foods, that's great. I just wish to emphasise that it is OK to eat the fuels that you feel really drawn to, as it is your body instructing you to fill up on the fuel that works.

So please relax into knowing that you should already be holding all the nutrition you and your developing embryo/foetus need.

The important time to be very concerned about nutrition comes around the 10–12 week mark. All through the second and third trimesters, nutrition is vital to the development of the foetus. At this time you must ensure that you are eating the best possible wholefoods with the highest possible nutrition to nurture that growing foetus.

Thankfully, as the placenta comes into full formation the pregnancy nausea should resolve. This is different for every woman, but this particular hormonal-soup nausea is usually something that only affects the first trimester.

If you are one of the unlucky women who really struggle with food and fluid input in the first trimester, you must please seek medical advice with your GP/midwife/obstetrician/local hospital antenatal outpatient unit. You must ensure that you remain hydrated: food and fluid depletion should always be monitored by qualified medical practitioners.

When it is too hard to get your antenatal supplement down, or you are vomiting a great deal, or struggle to take fluids, then please seek the advice of a good nutritionist who specialises in pregnancy and is adept at helping support women with these kinds of difficulties.

Lovemaking in the first trimester

This is simple, really – do you *fancy* a shag?

Then, yes!

So many women feel very protective of their bodies in this time, and in the context of this being such a hard-won conception, they often do not wish to do anything that may endanger the stability of the pregnancy.

Fair enough. The only thing you need to answer to is your own intuition. Often, our body feels so preoccupied that there really isn't any time or space for sexuality.

Often, it may be that you are in the throes of recovering from an IVF, and in this case I would advocate that it is important to not disturb the environment, for a big part of the construction in the case of an IVF conception is clearing up the site at the same time that all the new foundations are going in.

Sometimes the chemical soup can bring on a randiness like you haven't ever felt before, and you may find yourself all fired up and can't get enough. Fine, actually great! Fizz Maximus.

Even in the context of IVF tenderness, if your body is randy, then listen to what it is asking you for. Your intuition will tell you exactly what works, and you will find the positions that provide you with the safety and comfort to enjoy your sexuality. However, in the first few weeks of implantation, vigorous sex is not necessarily the best thing, for you do not want to disturb the uterus. This is a time when the womb needs to establish the vessel networks that will create the placenta.

Listen to your body. Move with intuition. If something is causing discomfort, ache or pain then simply change the position or stop. Sexuality during early pregnancy is entirely an intuitive process and trusting your body to show you what works is the best way to stay within entirely safe parameters.

Loving is Good! Follow your body's needs.

So we come back to the oxytocin message. Tenderness, cherishment, loving touch, stroking, massages, kissing and cuddling are so important. And girls, we do need to remember that though our bodies are going through these extraordinary shifts and changes, 12 weeks is a long time for guys to not receive the loving that their sabre craves. Hand jobs and blow jobs are a good way to stay connected sexually, and you can easily do that while being pregnantly horizontal!

The biology of the first trimester

The most important aspect of understanding the biology, is remembering that an embryo that arrests before 12 weeks does not hold the entire DNA map that will allow the development of embryo to foetus, to baby, to person.

As hard as it is, we must always bow to nature's law, and to respect that first trimester miscarriage is a normal part of the physiology of pregnancy. This is the *arrest* of an embryo and *not* the death of a baby.

Of course we must mourn, for we must grieve for the loss of the opportunity to become parents, for the loss of welcoming a child into our lives, for the loss of what might have been.

All of this needs to be processed. What is most important is to recognise that it is not a specific person who has been lost, but the potential for that person which has stopped.

If nature's laws dictate that this must be a pregnancy loss, you must reach deep inside yourselves to find the resilience that comes from recognising that you *can* get pregnant. You must keep that innermost part of your heart open to the possibility that you will conceive again. Be sure to turn towards each other, not away. By shutting yourselves off from each other you will force a lockdown that will only need to be re-opened in order to bring you back into your free-flowing loving bond.

I experienced my parents' loss when my little sister died at birth, and I have had both a termination and a miscarriage myself, and in understanding how much these events can undermine our sense of self, I have dedicated my life's work to helping people to have and raise healthy babies. If you are feeling lost and alone in the devastation, please be assured that you are not alone. There is so much support out there. Seek, and the people you need will be there, to help you, and give you solace.

It is so important to find the rituals that will take you through the steps of your grief and anger and frustration and loneliness and fear, then into the sadness.

Grief is a process, and we must go through all of its stages.

And when you reach the sadness, you must find a way to draw a line under your experience and bravely step forward into the next phase, secure in the knowledge that your hearts are safe, that you and your partner are going to take the next step together, and to find the courage to either try, try, and try again, or perhaps, to find the courage to acknowledge that this, perhaps, is the end of your fertility journey.

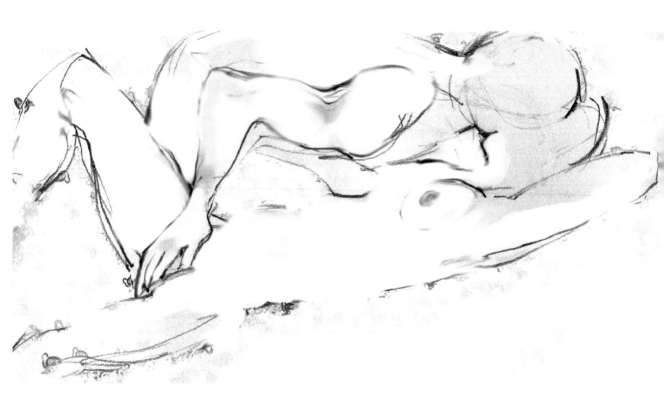

touch

such a wonderous thing
this anticipation
of a lover known, unknown

with words you open me
to the boundless possibilities
of allowing ourselves to be loving
unselfish

kindred we can share
and be in the glory of sexual expression
of the need to touch
the need to be touched

your finger
gently sliding on the slick of my juices
as you slowly slip the perimeter of my labia
ever widening circles
brushing open the pink of me

and my legs widen with your touch
my vulva swelling with the excitement of
the sweep of your probing strokes
pearlescent juice glistening an invitation to delve

come deeper my lover
find your way
towards the mysterious heart of me
feel the silky enticement of my flesh as i open wider
to your questing gypsy fingers

let my catching breaths fill you with
a fire to hear me ragged
as you begin exploratory descent into my cavernous delight
my quivering a tremor
reflected in your fingertip

the gloss of my slick juices swirl with your fingers
as you dance a teasing walk
entering into me
enveloped in my softest place
and in this exquisite tumble of sensations
my thighs clamp down upon your questing hand
and my breath pants, searing with the ache in my core

and i bear down upon your hand
with the hot gush of my desire
a torrent of salty liquid waterfalling over you
its heat so surprising and unexpected
and with a thrust
you dive fully into me
your force throwing my legs wide again

now urgent
cascading your fingers all over through and in
my head thrown back
with abject delight
in the ravishment of your owning

and then, softly, so softly
you hear me gasp a 'please'
oh please
let me feel your hot mouth against my aching quim
let me feel you lick the very juices your fingers just swirled

let me feel the heat of the descent of your tongue as you dive into me
flicking, licking, lapping
your hot hot tongue delving deeper and deeper
the thrust of my pelvis grinding you into me

and i reach and grasp my fingers in your hair
drawing, demanding
bringing you up and out of me
that you might descend upon
my erect and waiting clit
pulsating with the need to be enclosed
within the grasp of your mouth

and with a shout
my exclamation of desire met
rises to the night sky
as upon the sun warmed stone
you suck and lick and finger me
devouring
delighted
to make me shake with the momentum of my cumming

driving me down upon this place of magic and ruin
you bring me to the shuddering of the release
of wave upon wave of my wanting fulfilled
satiated in this moment beneath the stars

and as you lift your juice slickened face
i rise to meet you and draw your head to mine
that i might lick luscious moisture from your lips
and kiss you deeply

tasting me in you

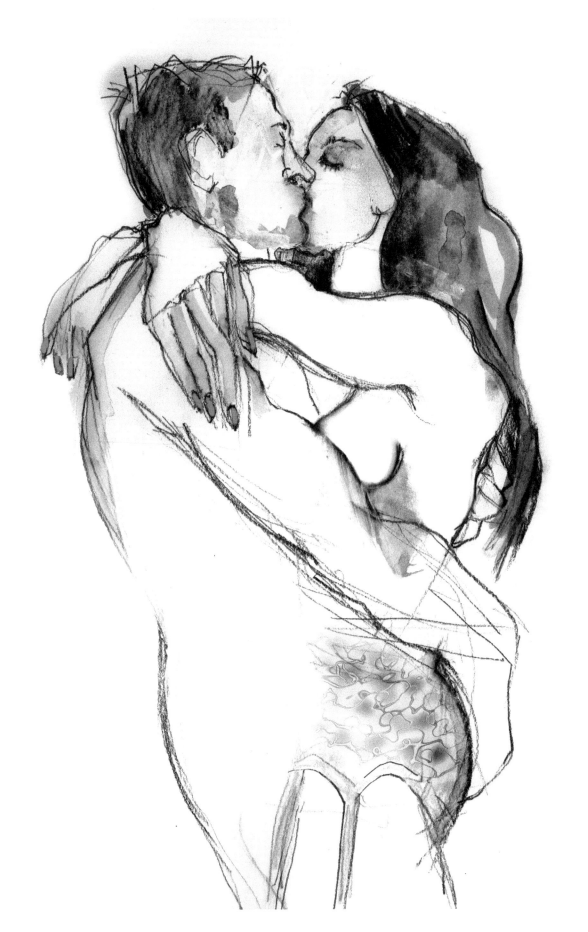

In Closing

Corridors

'Fertility journey' is an oft-repeated phrase, and for good reason. Anyone going through fertility issues is truly grappling with a very essential part of their self. The capacity to reproduce is hardwired within us and means that we do not choose our yearning for a child – it is part of our nature. We cannot choose to not feel it, it just is.

Journey – 'the act of travelling from one place to another'.

Synonyms: adventure, campaign, expedition, exploration, odyssey, passage, progress, quest ...

The fertility journey is like a long corridor, stretching for miles, and all the way along it there are doorways on each side. As we walk down this corridor it is important to open each of those doorways, to glimpse in and see if this is a room we need to enter and explore. Some of the rooms you do not actually need to go into, you can see at a glance that this is not for you. Others you need to step into, though you may find that you can deal with whatever it has to offer relatively quickly and return to the corridor.

Some rooms you need to step into and spend quite a bit of time there. There may be issues, physical or emotional, that you need to unpack and examine thoroughly.

Sometimes we might get stuck in a room and can't seem to find our way back into the corridor. Then you need to ask for help.

Sometimes we skip past a door and find we do need to double back to that unopened doorway.

As we make this journey, finding our way down this long, long corridor, we all the while have every one of our senses, mind and heart, attuned to the possibility that at the very end of this corridor there is that opportunity to have a baby, to become a family.

And sometimes we reach the end of that corridor, and there is no biological child to gather into our arms.

No one can say how long each corridor is, each one of us has a unique and individual journey. My wish is, when you do reach the end of your corridor, that you are able to turn around and look back down its length, seeing all those doorways, knowing a sense of peace in your heart, knowing that you did indeed explore each and every opportunity, delving into your psyche, delving into the biology, delving into the vulnerability, having given it your all.

May you stand at the end of that corridor and have no regrets. May you reach the end of this particular journey and know in your hearts that you did all that you could, no stone was left unturned, no doorway was passed by.

The journey of fertility will be an exploration of self, and it will also be an exploration of the relationship between you and your lover. And should you reach the end of that corridor finding that a biological child is not to be your gift, my wish is that your journey will have strengthened you both and your bond with each other, and that you may bravely make the next step into the life that awaits you beyond this corridor; that you may step out into a bright world that is filled with possibilities.

Should you not have the opportunity of birthing your own child, nor have a donor or surrogacy option, may you choose to fulfil your lives with a new purpose, directing your energies into whatever you wish to build and do, to nurture the next phase of your lives.

There are so many ways that we can step into our parenting energies.

Last words

I hope this book has been helpful. My ambition has been to help you connect to ideas that will resonate with you, to offer a resource from which you can cherry-pick the things that are most meaningful for you, and to help you find a way to Fizz up the sexuality that is at the very core of your capacity to conceive.

I want to empower you, to inspire you, to make you laugh and to reconnect you with feeling delight in your sexuality.

There are a hundred other things I would love to share, but it seems I have now used up my entire quota of exclamation marks ! & CAPITAL LETTERS & red & **bold** & *italics.*

Now is the right space and place to acknowledge all of the couples who I have ever worked with throughout the years – I have learned something from each and every one of you; and to all of the peer support with practitioners who have shared their clinical experiences, ever the most amazing learning curve a girl could hope for: and to all the learned teachers, both Western and Chinese medicine practitioners, who I have worked with who have so generously shared their wisdoms.

To all those TTC couples – your stories, your truths, your anguishes and your joys are the driver of this book.

Without your open-hearted sharing I could never have put all these words together.

These are your words, not mine.

I very much hope that these shared thoughts, ideas, suggestions, these 'sexy biology lessons' will somehow ease you on your journey, giving you a clearer sense of the totality of how our bodies work, recognising that we are what we think, we are what we eat, and that making babies is something we do with the whole of us – our hearts, our minds, our bodies.

I sincerely hope that the poetry and pictures have fed into the hot tips, and that you may feel more empowered to sail forth into an exciting reawakened exploration of your sexuality.

Get your freak on, find your turn on, sex it up and seduce your lover.
It's fun! (I saved one)

The chemistry of attraction *is* the chemistry of conception.

Happy lovemaking makes happy babies, for even if they happen to be fertilised in a petri dish, they are still being made inside of you, within all the love that you share.

So chill that bottle of bubbly … and when you do conceive, receive, donor, adopt, foster, make sure there is one in the fridge for when that longed for day arrives and your longed for person comes into your lives, however that might happen.

Wish for the child who needs you.

X jw

He whispered to her in the darkness as they lay together,

'Tell me where to touch you so that I can drive you insane ... tell me where to touch you to give you ultimate pleasure ... tell me where to touch you so that we will truly own each other'...

... She kissed him softly and whispered back,

'Touch my mind.'

~ Author Unknown

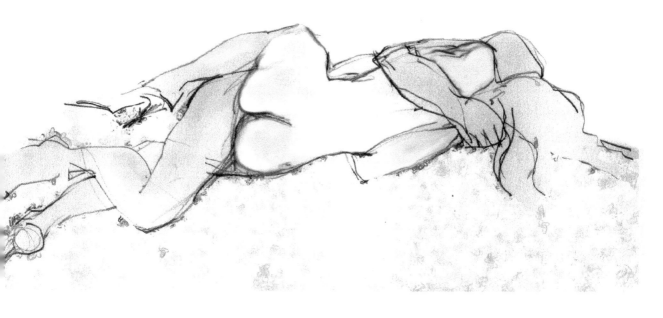

Index of illustrations

http://carolyn-weltman.pixels.com/

Index

References

Chapter Two

Alain de Botton, *How to Think More about Sex* (Macmillan, 2012): *www.theschooloflife.com/shop/how-to-think-more-about-sex/*

Chapter Four

www.babymad.com

Chapter Six

INUK (Infertility Network UK) has a very useful fact sheet about taking time off during an IVF cycle: *http://www.infertilitynetworkuk.com/uploaded/Fact%20 Sheets/Employment%20Time%20Off%20for%20 Fertility%20Treatment.pdf.*

Chapter Eight

Ashley Moffat, Lesley Regan and Peter Braude, *Natural killer cells, miscarriage, and infertility,* British Medical Journal, November 2004. *www.ncbi.nlm.nih. gov/pmc/articles/PMC534451/#!po=16.6667*

HFEA (Human Fertilisation and Embryology Authority).*www.hfea.gov.uk/fertility-treatment-options-reproductive-immunology.html#1*

www.helpguide.org/mental/emotional_psychological_ trauma.htm

The NHS has an excellent support system called PALS, the Patient Advice and Liaison Service: *www. nhs.uk/Service-Search/Patient-advice-and-liaison-services-(PALS)/LocationSearch/363)*

Chapter Eleven

Diagram of the Circadian rhythms. From Environmental Health Perspectives 2010 Jan; Vol 118; 1. Adapted by Matthew Ray/EHP.

Chapter Fourteen

Diagram of the dynamics of follicular growth. From Human Reproduction 1986 Feb; 1(2):81–7. *Dynamics of follicular growth in the human: a model from preliminary results.* Gougeon, A.

American Psychological Association: www.apa.org

British Psychology Society: www.bps.org.uk

Surrogacy UK: www.surrogacyuk.org/

The Infertility Network, INUK, have a website called More to Life: *www.infertilitynetworkuk.com/moretolife/*

Chapter Seventeen

www.nhs.uk/chq/Pages/how-can-i-work-out-my-bmi. aspx?CategoryID=51

Chapter Eighteen

Chavvaro & Willett, *The Fertility Diet* (McGraw Hill, 2008)

The Nurses Health Study Number 2 in 1989 *www.channing.harvard.edu/nhs/?page_id=70*

Coffee withdrawal symptoms: *http://coffeetea.about.com/od/caffeinehealth/a/Caffeine-Withdrawal-Symptoms.htm*

The caffeine milligram content in tea, coffee, chocolate and sodas: *http://infertility.about.com/od/ researchandstudies/a/caffeine_fertility.htm*

National Institute on Alcohol Abuse and Alcoholism: *www.niaaa.nih.gov/*

Appendix A

charting the menstrual cycle

For an in-depth discussion of all the following information, please listen to this Fertility Friday podcast:

http://www.fertilityfriday.com/janiwhite/

What follows is the series of questions that will help to determine a synopsis of the history and 'character' of your period:

When was Menarche? (age of first period)

How long did it take for the cycle to regulate?
*   When did you start using birth control?
*   Was this for sexual purposes, or was it prescribed to control your menstrual symptoms?

What was the length of the cycle (how many days eg: 28) and the character of the bleed in:
*   teens
*   20s
*   30s
*   present

We are interested to understand if it was different or the same during these different ages.

Also please note if there is a difference between how the cycle length and character behaves when you are on birth control or not.

Irregular cycle, meaning the whole cycle length:
*   too short
*   too long
*   no pattern
*   no periods

Irregular ovulation:
*   ascertained through BBT charting, use of ovulation predictor kits and by judging timing of cervical mucus.

Length of bleed:
*   1–2 days
*   2–3 days
*   3–4 days
*   4–5 days
*   5–7 days
*   longer?
*   varies, no discernable pattern

Quality of the bleed:
*   Scanty flow
*   heavy flow
*   Stop/Start flow

- regular medium-robust
- medium light

Colour of blood:
- regular ruby-red
- too dark
- too light
- watery
- bright blood

Clotted blood:
- liverish (looks like actual liver)
- stringy (looks like membranes)
- large or small?
- profuse or minimal?
- on which days of the bleed
- is there pain associated to the movement of a clot?

Cervical mucus:
- dry whitish discharge in the days after the period?
- changing to wet for a few days?
- slippery 'egg white' stretchy mucus just before ovulation?
- 'cheesy' or 'crumbly' luteal mucus after ovulation?

Inappropriate vaginal discharge?
- when?
- odour?
- colour
- amount?

Is there any pain?
- Region is significant, where is it?
- always in the same place, or does it move?
- in front or in the back? Or both?
- does it move from front to back, or move from back to front?
- at which point in the cycle?

- ovulatory?
- pre-menstrual?
- both?
- are there any mid-cycle sensations/tenderness/discomfort: called 'mittleschmerz'

When is the pain during the cycle:
- phase 1 – menstrual
- phase 2 – pre ovulation
- during ovulation
- phase 3 – post ovulation
- phase 4 – pre-menstrual

Describe the quality of the pain:
- any words that accurately describes what you are feeling
- constant
- come and go
- gripping
- knifing
- drilling
- squeezing
- twisting
- stabbing
- dull ache
- pressing ache

What eases the menstrual pain:
- do you want to curl up and apply a hot water bottle?
- does the pain ease if you do stretching exercise such as yoga
- does the pain clear with vigorous walking or running?

Contraception history:
- what kind/s of birth control have you used at which ages?
- For how long? In what order?
- How have the periods behaved since coming off?

– the contraceptive pill
– the morning after pill
– cap/diaphragm with spermicidal gels
– condoms with spermicidal gels
– the coil / Mirena coil
– hormone patches / injections / implant
– termination

Miscarriage or termination:
- has this left any emotional scars for you?
- did this change the character of the periods?

Is there any history of:
- accidents
- injuries
- surgeries
- trauma – emotional or physical
- any bereavements or grief

Signs & Symptoms checklist for before and during the period:

When does PMS begin – how many days post ovulation? Are there any PMS symptoms at ovulation? Is there a pattern, or does it change with each cycle?

- Breast changes
  – sore sides
  – sore in the body of the breast
  – sore nipples
  – heavy and uncomfortable
- Water retention
- Abdominal changes / bloating
- Appetite changes / cravings / aversions
- Bowel movements – stool quality / frequency / constipation
- Urinary changes
- Sleep pattern changes
- Headache – where, when and how

- dizziness / floaters (black dots in your vision)
- sweating / night sweats / flushes
- emotional lability
  – short tempered / intolerant
  – feeling angry – either pent up or lashing out
  – frustration
  – feeling oversensitive with a tendency to cry
  – overly emotional / over-reacting
- bruise easily
- clumsiness
- memory problems
- lack of libido
- overly randy (raging libido)

Chinese medicine for menstrual regulation

These notes should give you a greater sense of how Chinese medicine practitioners gather and collate your menstrual history, signs & symptoms.

All of this information will help to give your practitioner a much better understanding of the bespoke treatment that would be used to help regulate your cycle.

Even if you are not seeing a Chinese medicine practitioner, by taking all of these notes into consideration you will greatly improve your charting skills.

Learning to observe each of your phases will help you to become very aware of your cycle – not only for while you are trying to conceive, but for the future as well, for all ages and all stages.

This is your womanly self.

Taking care of our menstrual cycle is a deep part of how we can care for our self.

Appendix B

supplementary BBT charting notes

Monitoring the cycle rhythms with BBT, LH surge and signs & symptoms observation

Your BBT chart should act as much more than a temperature record, it should become a really useful diary that helps you to learn to understand your cycle, to help you develop a strong and clear sense of your body's fluctuations, and to learn how these fluctuations affect your libido.

See chapter Four

Adjusting your Chart when you have a lie-in:

I always suggest choosing the most regular time that you need to get up for work – BUT – when it comes to weekends it's important for your REST to be able to wake naturally rather than to an alarm. There is a simple way that you can adjust the temp reading, to allow that lie-in, but still have a clear record of the rhythms of your cycle.

To adjust your temperature according to the time there is a simple formula (based in centigrade measurement). For every half hour you adjust the temperature by 1/10th of a degree.

So if you usual time is 7 a.m., when you sleep later you bring the temperature back down, and if you wake earlier you bring the temperature back up. I was confused by this at first until I learned a simple way to calculate the adjustment.

Hold your hands up in front of you to mark your usual median time, say 7 a.m. If you sleep in until 9, then move your hands up to count the half hours: 7:30, 8, 8:30, 9 = 4/10ths. So your hands have moved upwards, therefore you know you need to **subtract** in order to come back **down** to your median time.

So when you are recording the adjusted temperature mark it in 4/10th below the time on the thermometer.

If you wake earlier, say 5:30 (yuck, commonly known as 'stupid o'clock in our house'), then you need to move your hands downwards, 6:30, 6, 5:30 = 3/10ths. So you now need to move your hands upwards to come back to your median time, therefore you need to **add** that 3/10ths of a degree in order to come back **up** to your median line.

Always note the time when you take your temperature.

It is really helpful to mark in the recorded temperature at the time you have actually taken it, and then to mark in the adjusted temperature as well. When you join the dots to make the picture of the pattern be sure to join the line to the adjusted temp. This will give a more accurate picture and still allow you the leisure and rest and benefits of having a sleep-in.

This is one of the reasons I prefer to have a written record rather than an electronic one.

If you are using a charting app then please always record the adjusted temperature, so as to generate the most accurate pattern when the lines are drawn to connect the dots.

Always apply notes about any significant events ie: late nights, alcohol intake, travel, change of diet, sleep disruption, etc. …

The more detail you apply to your charting, the more you will learn about how your lifestyle affects your period throughout every phase of the cycle.

Happy charting!

Appendix C

Men's sexual health

Timing sex when you are trying to conceive

Frequency of intercourse should be based on the consideration of:
- strength of constitution (overall health + genetic tendencies)
- age
- season of the year
- sperm parameter measures

A range of 1–5 times per week is normal.

These signs and symptoms may suggest that the sexual energy reserves are low:
- fatigue (meaning: always feeling tired on waking in the mornings/low energy throughout the day)
- weakness of the lower back and the knees
- decreased frequency of morning erections
- decreased firmness of erections
- decreased orgasmic intensity

These signs are barometers for detecting that the sexual drive is compromised and may suggest a need to reduce sexual frequency.

Sperm parameters:
- If the concentration is low, meaning less than 20 ml/ml, then it is advised to have sexual intercourse with a minimum of 48 hours between lovemaking during the fertile time.
- This allows the concentration to build back up to peak for each ejaculate.

A sysnopsis of issues that degrade sexual health:

Overwork and dietary irregularities are endemic in Western society:
- It is common for work to encompass full time plus evenings plus weekends
- Commuting time should be accounted as a taxation
- Domestic responsibilities have increased with higher expectation of house maintenance and childcare, so many responsibilities!
- Overwork often comes with:
  – Erratic eating schedule
  – Scanty or no breakfast, ie: coffee and pastry
  – Skipping lunch or grabbing a sandwich in front of the computer
  – Eating too much, too rich, too late in the evening
- Grab and go diet leads to decreased libido, to decreased fertility and to 'yang wilt'.

Useful Resources

I would especially like to recommend the books by my colleague Jill Blakeway. Her wise words, her calm and deep knowledge, imbibe both of these volumes with wonderful advice and guidance. I think these are a perfect accompaniment to *The Fertile Fizz*.

Links to both Jill Blakeway's books, *Making Babies* and *Sex Again* can be found here:

https://jillblakeway.com/

The Amazon link, to both books, is:

http://www.amazon.co.uk/s/ref=nb_sb_noss_2/278-7470368-3892130?url=search-alias%3Daps&field-keywords=Jill%20blakeway

Another wonderful writer to discover is Julia Indichova. Her website is a font of wonderful positive support: http://www.fertileheart.com/

Both of Julia's books, *Inconceivable* and *The Fertile Female* sit alongside Fizz as ideal companions. Follow this link to source these books:

http://www.fertileheart.com/shop/bookshelf/from-fertile-heart/

Although many of the sites I am recommending are UK based, they are full of solid advice, useful no matter where you are. These sites necessarily may advocate UK standards, procedures and protocols. They may also help guide you to similar sites in your own countries …

Fertility Awareness

http://www.fertilityfriday.com/

Infertility Network UK – full of wonderful advice

http://www.infertilitynetworkuk.com/

Fertility Friends – a forum for TTC couples

http://www.fertilityfriends.co.uk/

HFEA – the Human Fertilisation Embryo Authority

http://www.hfea.gov.uk/

One at a Time – multiple birth

http://www.oneatatime.org.uk/

DC Network – Donor Conception Network

http://www.dcnetwork.org/

Surrogacy

http://www.surrogacyuk.org/

Women's Sexuality – this is brilliant!

https://www.omgyes.com/

Men's Sexual and Reproductive Health

http://theturekclinic.com/blog/

Pregnancy Loss & Bereavement – You are not alone

www.childbereavement.org.uk
www.babyloss-awareness.org
www.winstonswish.org.uk
www.childdeathhelpline.org.uk

British Acupuncture Council – the professional body for Traditional Acupuncture in the UK

https://www.acupuncture.org.uk/

Acupuncture Fertility Network – UK

http://www.acupuncture-fertility.org/

American Board of Oriental Medicine – USA

http://aborm.org/

In Respect of Erotic Exploration – the Internet is Your Oyster!

Here are a few sites about finding guidance to explore intimacy and erotic boundaries and will help give you an idea of what is out there …

http://www.drewlawson.co/
http://www.eroticeducation.org/
https://www.kinkly.com/
http://mytinysecrets.com
http://www.seanilove.com/

There is now a fast-growing trend of qualified sexual therapists who are there to help support you to finding safe ways to explore your intimacy, your pleasures and your willingness to adventure. They are far too many to mention, and looking for the right one in your area can be half the fun!

We are always interested to find quality sites that have impressed you, so please feel free to email us any suggestions of sites we should see:

connect@fertilefizz.com

Glossary

Though I grew up in Canada, I moved to England three decades ago and I now consider myself to be bilingual.

This book is peppered with English idioms and language, so, for those who may not know what some of these funny words are, this is for you … X jw

'England and America are two countries
separated by a common language.'

George Bernard Shaw

flummoxed = bewildered or perplexed

knackered = **tired**, like *really* tired, as in a horse no longer able to stand (in a pre-car world) who is taken to the 'knackers' yard where they would be put down

cream crackered = **knackered** cockney rhyming slang (look it up)

knickers = **panties,** girl's underwear, undies, drawers, cheekies, briefs, butt huggers, boy shorts, thongs, g-strings, tighty whities, skivvies, drawers, underpants, undergarments, underthings, *lingerie*!

NB - in the UK **pants = boy's underwear**. Much snickering when our American friends go out in their pants rather than putting on their trousers
Urban dictionary says: '**pants = rubbish**, no good, bag of shite' (I quote)

bollocks = rubbish
Urban Dictionary : 'a highly flexible term commonly used by the English'
1. something rubbish *something pants*
2. a falsehood or series of lies *'he's talking bollocks'*
3. something great *'the dogs bollocks'*
4. the best possible *erhm, because dogs can lick their own ...*
5. testicles *testicles*
6. exclamation on making a error *(can be used interchangeably with 'oh, Bugger!' in these circumstances)*

rubbish = trash
bin = trash can

bonkers = crazy, as in driving me ...

shag = having sex
bonking = having sex not to be confused with bonkers
nookie = having sex
morning glory = morning wood
gee up / geeing = get excited
your wheeze = whatever turns you on can be used both sexually and non-sexually, not to be confused with emphysema

wee = small as in ***wee bairn* = small baby** said in a Scottish accent

cuppa = cup of tea the great British medicinal remedy for all ills and woes

tuck = treats usually meaning **sweets = candy** a hangover word from English **Public Schools = private schools** as opposed to **state schools = public schools**

like the (berloody) **clappers = go very fast in a vigorous manner** derived from English public schoolboys (see above) having to run to class as bells were rung – did you know that hand bells have clappers – and the nearer to the starting time of class or **chapel = church** the more vigorously the bells would ring and more vigorously the boys would run

berloody = the politer form of bloody from an era when bloody was considered a vulgar swear word

hammer and tongs = energetically and enthusiastically – a fabulous way to have sex – *'they were going at it hammer and tongs'*

rate of knots = doing something very quickly a naval term to measure the speed a boat travels, back in the day when a sailing ship was the fastest thing on earth. Really

eww-err-missus = gosh, ain't that grand, a West Country (Somerset, Devon, Cornwall) working-class expression, predominantly agricultural

grand = wonderful

womb = common parlance for uterus
uterus - the medical term for womb

<u>ante</u>natal = <u>pre</u>natal Latin: *ante* meaning before, *natal* meaning birth
intrapartum = during labour
post partum = after labour

Tube = London Underground the subway system in the capital, subterranean hell in rush hour

lorry = truck
petrol = gasoline

maths = arithmetic
marker (pen) = felt tip
nursery = childcare / day care / preschool

chat show = talk show

Unit = IVF Clinic where you go to have assisted conception, many IVF clinics here in the UK are based in hospitals, hence the term 'unit' as a part of the hospital.

NHS = National Health Service a most marvellous institution for public health that is on its knees and wheezing (as in emphysema), and is an institution to be proud of even in the context of its bureaucratic failings. We love the NHS for all it does do, ever against these incredible political odds

HFEA = Human Fertilisation Embryo Authority the body that governs all aspects of the practice of Assisted Conception in the UK. I can't find any way to take the piss, they are a good, even handed governmental body that manage the regulations in the context of both UK and EU (European Union) guidelines and directives

take the piss = to mock someone/something another great British institution

Tesco/Sainsbury's = Safeway/Aldi/Trader Joe's the big supermarket chains that dominate the field

slay the woolly mammoth = bring home the bacon meaning our trip round the aisles with a **shopping trolley = grocery cart** is equivalent to our hunter-gather ancestors fight to survive by bringing home all sustenance in one go. So grateful to not have to skin and butcher one of those!

charity shops = goodwill store where most of my clothes come from, in the UK supporting charity shops is cool

cheap as chips = not at all expensive and why the Brits like to support charity shops

old money = pounds, shillings and pence as opposed to new money which is decimalised. Slang for an old system which is no longer in use. Whatever will I do with all my ha'pennies? (pronounced hay-penny)

cheerio = goodbye, but will see you again a bit like the difference between *adieu* (not sure when we'll see each other again) and *au revoir* (until next time)

The Artist

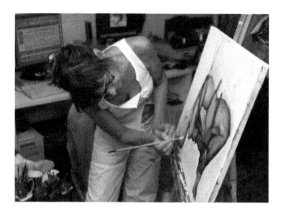

'Carolyn Weltman declares herself an expressive figurative artist whose work includes female, male, transgender and transitioning subjects. Her portrayal of sexually aggressive figures bound and in flight is unmatched, whatever the gender. Her work is full of wonder …'

The characters in my paintings and drawings are powerful and made only more so for enduring how I would portray them. Consider the throbbing kinesis of a body captured in bondage, and compare to it the exuberant trajectories of the trapeze artist, glorious dancers in air. Draw them both into the perfectly disciplined stop-motions of the danseuse or the athlete. Sense all of it in the break of a fallen boxer's breath as taut muscles pause to reignite. All slices of stilled, economical motion, exploring the inner idea, the corporeal feeling, and the outer expression, all outside of time.

My intention is to bring you, the viewer, into that slice, into the exploration, and out of time. In the end my work is about acceptance of self and other. And even self as other. The more of one's senses are engaged and the higher their vibration (and the erotic is nothing if not a sensation-amplifier) the closer one skirts the transcendent. Art elevates as it breaks down division and presses towards unity, and the erotic is all about getting us to that principle of unity as expeditiously and as often as possible. I draw the human form in uncommon states, for it falls to a body to embody us in the first place, and to our bodies to carry us all, finally, out. Within the small time slice of our lives our bodies, along with our minds and our souls, deserve our honour.

http://www.artforengineers.com

The Poet

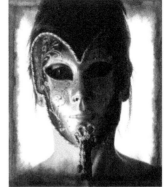

In this book, between each section, for your delectation, we have shared with you the 'Erotic Musings of Rebecca Deacon', whose poetry is her personal experience of the unfolding discovery of her deepest sexual self.

Though she feels shy about having these soul-baring most intimate words put to print, she feels that the erotisicm of her experience is something she would like to share; this is her journey of discovery into the darkest corners of her longings. With great generosity, she has given her words to this book.

These extracts are mostly drawn from the correspondence of Rebecca and her lover, 'The Gypsy Pirate' who lives far far away in Another Country.

They connected on the Internet, and from the very first message they both felt that something unique and tantalising and compelling was afoot.

They immediately tumbled into a racy exchange, and within days it was clear they would need to meet. She jumped on a plane and never looked back – stepping into one of the Great Adventures of her life.

The ensuing months and years have unfolded a truly erotic connection of lust and love and an enduring friendship.

The Writer

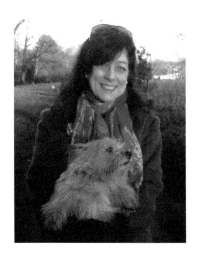

Jani is a highly experienced acupuncturist, she lectures nationally and internationally in her subjects, as well as having many years experience in all aspects of childbirth.

Jani's specialities are wide ranging, though the core of her work is in one pillar – the Endocrine System – your hormones. She treats all ages, both male and female, infant to geriatric and everyone in between.

Jani treats in a fully integrative capacity, blending the best of Western and Chinese medicine, always with the agenda to ensure that her patients will receive the right combination of investigations and treatments, in the right sequence, to bring the best possible solutions in the most efficient way.

Jani came to Chinese medicine through her own illness, and a very amazing 'miracle cure' experience that set her on the path of studying this medicine. She really loves the privilege of being able to answer her vocational passion for teaching, ever only the senior learner, and enjoys this aspect of her work more than anything.

Uhhmmm, Errr, wait a sec! But isn't being a doula the very favourite part of her work? Yes indeed. For there is nothing she loves more than to help facilitate a gentle and joyful physiologic birth. Well there is actually, Jani's idea of a perfect birth is being with a couple who originally came for fertility treatment and she is able to be there when the baby is born. Sublime!

And she absolutely loves being in clinic, almost as much as she loves being able to write about all the things which she feels such passion for. Watch for the next 4 titles in this 5-part series ... Next up, *Birth-fit Fizz*.

Jani considers herself to be most fortunate indeed, to 'live her work – not work to live', and to have such a rich world filled with multitudes of really excellent people, and so many colleagues and patients who also become friends. Every day she thanks her lucky stars.

www.janiwhite.com (social) and (clinic) www.acuhouse.co.uk

Acknowledgements

You know that thing? The bit where the writer makes that ever-constant comment – '...my amazing publishers...' Well – it's my turn. I never realised when I embarked on this just why every writer on the planet feels compelled to write this acknowledgement – and now I do.

Clare Christian, the moment I saw your Red Door, I knew I needed to step through it. Thank you for instantly having faith in this project, and for the stellar guidance that has led to this publication.

Heather Boisseau, Book-Doula Extraordinaire. Your calm clear handholding has made this whole incredible birthing a wonderful experience. Thank you for seeing my vision and making it manifest, all the while helping me to do it my way. That's what really good Doulas do.

Sadie Mayne, Editor with a razor sharp touch, you slashed my verbosity to shreds and allowed the voice to remain. Thank you for taking such good care of the words, and for losing the plethora of exclamation marks.

To all the Team who made this book possible. Your ability to take on board what we are creating, a whole new format, has given me peaceful sleeps knowing your skills were engineering the pages that would delight the reader.

Typesetter: **Megan Sheer**. Proofreader: **Kathy Steer.** Indexer: **Lisa Footit.** Cover Design: **Clare Turner**

Tarka Sands, who knew that a ginger-intro (Thanks Olivia!) would lead to a dj'ing logo designer named after an otter. My delight knows no bounds, it is sheer pleasure to work with you.

And to my Kickstarters... (who kicked my butt)

Vincent Rowley, who makes making videos so much fun. 'Pithy Darling, Keep It Pithy!' Your unfailing support for this project is deep in the core of our friendship. Thank you for making it all so fun & sexy.

Mo Fine, who had the bright idea to endlessly bombard all my friends & family, colleagues, patients and acquaintances through 30 hair-raising days of watching the total trickle then flow then flood. Thank you Mo for making this happen. It was a good idea.

Caroline Muzio, Our First Pledge, who tweeted up a Fertile Storm. Your faith in this project has been a magnificent support, you are foundation to making this happen. Thank You.

I most especially wish to thank

Dr Debra Betts,

who encouraged this book into being. She expressed her faith in me, a compliment so great; and whilst rambling with the dogs along the Oxfordshire Thames riverside one fine English summer's day, in a tumble of conversation on the way to a pub lunch, she gave this book its title.

Dr Lorne Brown,

first in Rothenburg, under a star lit sky outside the Zur Hoell tavern, then again in Nottingham in 'the oldest pub in England', it is because of you that this has become an actual book.

Dr Jane Lyttleton,

who inspired me like no other, whose teaching has been so foundation to my work, and whose friendship and guidance has shaped my practice. It is your work that imbibes into mine to every one of my fertility patients.

X jw